THE COMPLETE GUIDE TO ESSENTIAL OILS

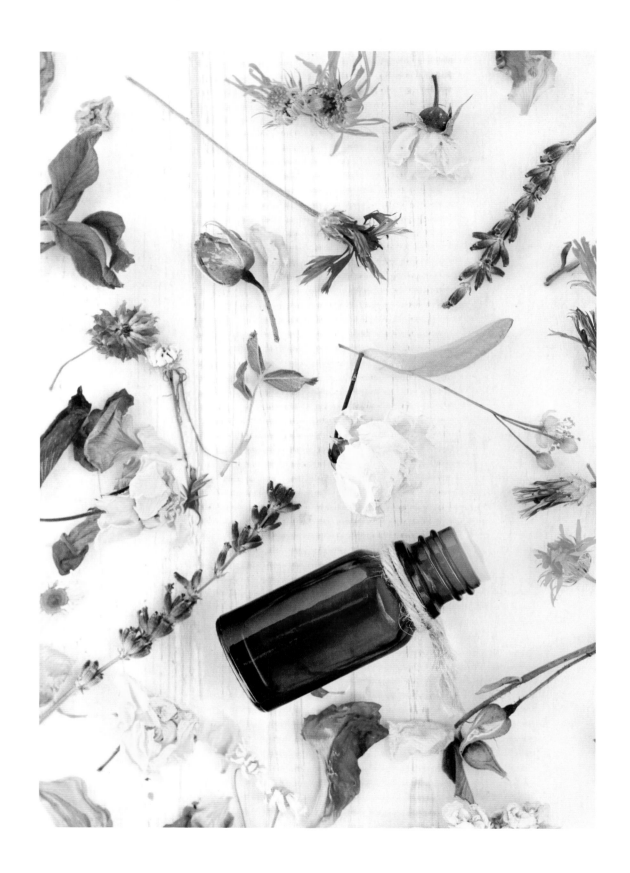

THE COMPLETE GUIDE TO ESSENTIAL OILS

How to use essential oils for health,
beauty, and well-being

GILL FARRER-HALLS

ISBN: 978-0-85762-885-5

QTT:EOIL

Conceived, designed, and produced by:
The Bright Press, an imprint of The Quarto Group,
6 Blundell Street,
London, N7 9BH
United Kingdom
T (0)20 7700 6700 F (0)20 7700 8066
www.quartoknows.com

Project Editors: Jessica Cowie, Cara Frost-Sharratt,
Leah Feltham
Designers: Tania Gomes, Tokiko Morishima,
Marie Boulanger
Picture research: Lauren Azor
Editorial Director: Emma Bastow
Publisher: Mark Searle

Printed in China by Toppan Leefung

2 4 6 8 10 9 7 5 3 1

This book is intended for educational purposes only
and is not a substitute for medical advice. Pregnant
and breastfeeding women, the elderly, and anyone
suffering from a serious illness should consult a
qualified healthcare professional before using essential
oils. Always read the information provided before use,
and note that some oils are not suitable for use on
babies and children.

Essential oils should be stored out of reach of children
and pets. Avoid contact with the eyes; consult a
medical professional immediately if contact occurs.
Some oils can cause skin irritation, and it is advised
that those with sensitive skin perform a patch test 24
hours before use. The ingestion of essential oils is not
advised except where indicated.

Image Credits

t = top, b = bottom, l = left, r = right,
m = middle

Alamy: Tim Gainey 69bl; Phanie 69br, 72br; Avalon/
Photoshot License 132; D. Hurst 142bl; Art of
Nature 157

Getty Images: Anna-Ok 2; MacoMarchi 6t; JGI/
Jamie Grill 6bl; Russell Sadur 9; 5second 11tl;
ChamilleWhite 13, 103; Bernard Radvaner/Corbis
19; Albertem 21; Thuy Tran/EyeEm 29; Tier Und
Naturfotografie J und C Sohns 35; Milles Studio 37b;
Foxys_forest_manufacture 39bl; Nanthaphiphat_Watto
41; Kerrick 50t; violetta 53; bunhill 63; Westend61
67; La_vanda 69t; sykono 71r; Garo/Phanie 72t;
Stieglitz 72bl; Victoria Pearson 79l; Erika McConnell
79r; simaric 83; Merethe Svarstad Eeg/EyeEm; 84t;
gehringj 91l; SondraP 92t; jennybonner 92bl; janaph
92br; Ignacio Palacios 95; Anne Hyde 97br; LazingBee
100t; hereswendy 100bl; Visuals Unlimited, Inc./David
Sieren 100br; Joan Ransley 105br; Flowerphotos/
Contributor 107; Maya23K 109; Rimma_Bondarenko
111; Coput 112t; YelenaYemchuk 117; Taka 119;
Bico_raro 123; microgen127; JohnnyGreig 129;
EasterBunnyUK 131; GlobalStock 135; Fran Gealer
137t; sorsillo 137b; jaminwell 141t; DavorLovincic
142br; James and James 143; Yannick Tylle 151;
fotomem 153; moodboard 155

Shutterstock: lizabarbiza 11bl; Antonova Ganna
25; janaph 27; Leonardo Da 33; Kerdkanno 39t;
spkphotostock 39bl; Todja 39mr; Artem Shadrin 42t;
VICUSCHKA 42bl, 49; SherSor 50bl; Fortforks 57t;
Hulia Sudnitskaya 64; Oleysa Baron 71l; Melpomene
77tl; Cindy Hughes 77tr; Shumytskyi Oleh 77mr;
images72 77b; Billion Photos 81b; MATHIR MOHD
YASIN 84br; NeydtStock 105t; Bozhena Melnyk 114;
BABAROGA 121; Dory F 144; Swapan Photography
149t; KatieKK 149b

Stocksy: Nataša Mandic 6br; Helen Rushbrook 11br;
Pixel Stories 14t; Jovana Rikalo 22ml; Juan Moyano
30; Mosuno 42br; Daniel Kim Photography 45; Zocky
57bl; Naoko Kakuta 57br; Dobránska Renáta 59;
Federica Di Marcello 61; Lumina 75, 81t, 147; Marilar
Irastorza 84bl; Rhonda Adkins 87l; Good Vibrations
Images 97t; Lyuba Burakova 97bl; Elessio Bogani
105bl; Nadine Greeff 125; Christine Han 139

Also: Lauren Azor 112

*While every effort has been made to credit photographers,
Quintet, an imprint of the Quarto Group, would like to
apologize should there have been any omissions or errors,
and would be pleased to make the appropriate correction
for future editions of the book.*

CONTENTS

INTRODUCTION 7

THE ESSENTIAL OILS

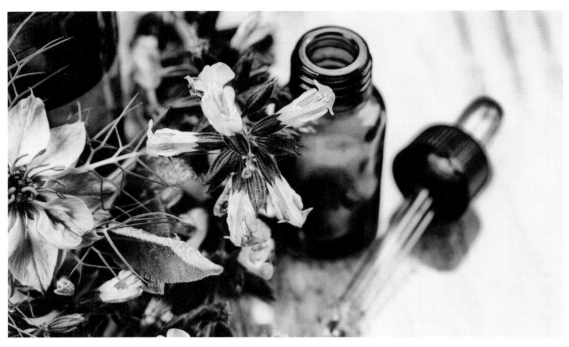

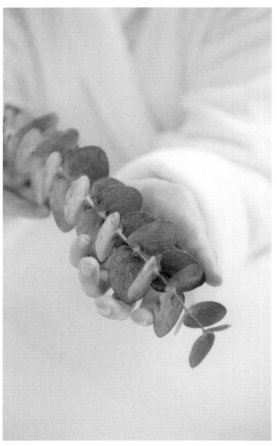

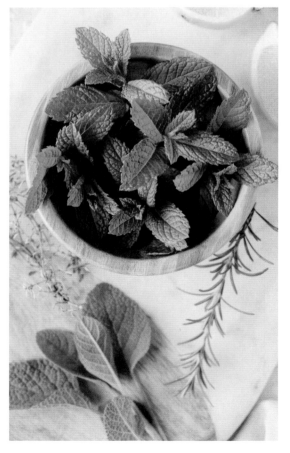

INTRODUCTION

Over the last few decades, essential oils have become increasingly popular. Some people have a regular or occasional aromatherapy massage, and many more also use essential oils in the bath, and in burners, creams, and lotions, and around the home. In this way essential oils provide natural alternatives to chemically based soaps, cleaners, detergents, and air fresheners.

This book for the general reader offers a simple introduction to a wide variety of essential oils, providing all the basic information you need, including how to use the oils effectively and safely. For each essential oil details are provided of the botanical family, method of extraction, fragrance description, and the therapeutic properties (you will find a glossary of terms on page 158). The profile of each essential oil also comes with a simple recipe, so you can create your own aromatherapy products using different essential oils and the plants and herbs from which they are extracted.

WHAT ARE ESSENTIAL OILS?

Essential oils are derived from naturally occurring aromatic essences within fragrant plants. These essences play an important role in nature, as they help aromatic plants thrive; the scents attract bees for pollination and repel predatory animals and insects. Not all plants are aromatic, but many are either fragrant or highly scented. Essential oils are derived from the parts of plants containing the aromatic essences—such as herbs, flowers, berries, seeds, grasses, and spices.

Naturally occurring plant essences have complex chemical structures based on the process of photosynthesis. This transforms the energy locked in sunlight and combines it with nutrients from air, water, and earth. Steam distillation is the most frequent method of extraction used to produce essential oil, but there are other methods such as simple expression of fruit rinds. This is something we can try at home—by squeezing orange peel we can extract a few drops of sweet orange essential oil. Although essential oils are technically oils and so do not dissolve in water, they are mostly clear, thin, and non-greasy.

To use essential oils safely, in most cases they should first be dissolved in carrier oils such as sweet almond oil, or alcohol. Essential oils are highly concentrated, meaning they are very powerful, which is why they are usually diluted before applying them to the skin. Essential oils are volatile, so they swiftly evaporate when exposed to the air. This is what gives them their perfuming ability, and why you should always put the cap on the bottle as soon as you have finished using it.

AROMATICS THROUGHOUT HISTORY

Essential oils were not readily available until steam distillation was discovered, probably by the Persian Avicenna in the 10th century. Nonetheless, plant aromatics played a significant role in ancient cultures. An important use of these early aromatics, and later on essential oils, was to please and pacify the gods. Incense and other aromatic preparations were burned so the fragrant smoke would ascend to the heavens and reach them. This supplication and fragrant offering was made to appease often wrathful deities, along with the hope of bringing good fortune and bountiful crops, and avoiding floods, plagues, and famines.

Aromatics were also offered to the gods in sacred rituals because they were expensive and highly prized. The valuable healing properties of burning aromatic herbs were discovered almost by accident when priests making sacred offerings noticed that breathing the smoke made them feel relaxed or invigorated, or even helped them recover from ailments. Individual ancient cultures had their own ways of using aromatics beyond the sacred. In ancient Egypt, Queen Cleopatra seduced Mark Anthony not with her beauty, but with her skill in perfumes and presentation. She sailed down the Nile to meet him in a ship with sails impregnated with rose oil, the most aphrodisiac—and costly—perfume.

The finest frankincense grew in ancient southwest Arabia. Together with other spices and aromatics, these were so highly valued that they were used as trading commodities. This gave Arabia significant trading and economic advantages, and this was still the case when Shakespeare wrote "the Scottish play" *Macbeth*. Lady Macbeth goes mad, and while sleepwalking utters the famous lines: "Here's the smell of blood still. All the perfumes of Arabia will not sweeten this little hand."

SAFETY

Essential oils are highly concentrated and can be dangerous if used incorrectly. This is easily demonstrated by the fact it takes thousands of jasmine petals to produce a single drop of jasmine. This potency must be respected, and it's important to handle essential oils correctly. By following the guidelines below, you can use essential oils safely and effectively.

- Never ingest essential oils orally unless they have been highly diluted, according to recipe instructions. It can be illegal for a qualified aromatherapist to suggest taking essential oils internally. Avoid all contact with mouth and eyes.

- Some essential oils can cause skin irritation if applied undiluted, so this is generally not recommended (with a few exceptions). Only apply properly diluted essential oils to the skin unless there are specific instructions otherwise.

- The profile of each essential oil indicates if it might cause skin irritation for those with sensitive skin. Occasionally, a slight redness or itchiness might occur from using these, or any essential oil. If this happens apply some base cream or carrier oil to the affected area, and place a cold, wet flannel on top until the symptoms disappear.

- Never increase the amount of essential oils used in recipes, and follow the instructions precisely.

- If you accidentally splash a drop of essential oil in your eyes, use a small amount of carrier oil to dilute the essential oil. Absorb the oils with a soft cloth before rinsing your eyes with cold water. Then seek urgent medical advice.

USING ESSENTIAL OILS

Aromatherapists offer massage to their clients, using a blend of essential oils in a carrier oil. However, for use at home the following methods are generally used.

- **Baths**
  You can add 3–6 drops of essential oil into the bath, but it is better to dilute the oils in base bath oil. Most of these are dispersant which creates a milky effect as the oils are dispersed in the water.

- **Steam inhalations**
  When you have a cold, sinusitis, or other respiratory ailment, steam inhalations with essential oils relieve symptoms and help you recover. Add 2–4 drops of a recommended essential oil to a bowl of boiling water. Place a towel over your head and, keeping your face a safe distance from the hot water, inhale the vapors for a few minutes.

- **Vaporizers and burners**
  Ceramic burners are easy to use. The base holds a tea-light candle and the bowl on top holds water and essential oil. Pour hot water into the bowl, light the candle, and float up to 8 drops of essential oil on the water. As the heat increases, the scent becomes stronger. Antiseptic and antiviral essential oils prevent the spread of infection, while any essential oil will fragrance your room. Vaporizers are electric and don't use water: the effect is similar to a burner.

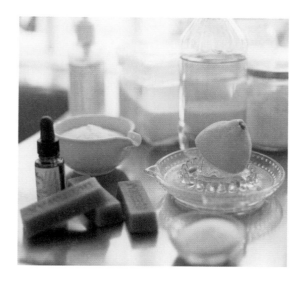

- **Perfumes and room fresheners**
  You can make simple roll-on oil perfumes using a ½ fl oz (10 ml) glass bottle with a rollerball insert. Half fill the bottle with jojoba oil and add a maximum of 20 drops of essential oil. Shake to mix the oils together, top up with jojoba and shake again before inserting the roller ball. For room fresheners you need a 3½ fl oz (100 ml) dark-glass spray bottle. Pour a little perfumer's alcohol (see page 40) into the bottle, add 20 drops of essential oil, and shake well. Top up with distilled water, and shake again.

- **Cold and hot compresses**
  Compresses using essential oils are good for first aid. Hot compresses over the kidneys and lower back are good for cystitis, while cold compresses relieve the pain and swelling of sprains and strains. Fill a bowl with either very hot water, or cold water and ice. Float 2–3 drops of the recommended essential oil on the surface; it will spread out into a fine film on top. Use a flannel to soak up the oil and some water and apply to the affected area. Repeat 2–3 times.

LAVENDER

Lavandula angustifolia 'Mill', Lavandula officinalis

Botanical Family:
Lamiaceae (Labiatae)

A popular traditional plant, lavender is a familiar sight in many gardens. In summer the bush produces long spikes with fragrant purple flowers on the tips.

METHOD OF EXTRACTION:
Lavender is steam distilled from the flowering tops, which include mainly the flower heads.

REGIONS OF ORIGIN:
Australia, Bulgaria, England, France, Hungary, Morocco, Spain, Tasmania.

CHARACTERISTICS:
Lavender is a clear, thin essential oil that easily drops from the bottle dropper.

FRAGRANCE DESCRIPTION:
Lavender has clean, fresh, floral top notes and subtle, green, herbaceous undertones. Usually described as a middle note in perfumery.

SAFE USAGE: Avoid in the first three months of pregnancy, especially if there is a history of miscarriage.

PLANT DESCRIPTION

The bush is often buzzing with insects, including bees, which visit to feast on the lavender flower nectar.

Several different varieties of lavender are now available, including alba, which has white flowers, and munstead, and hidcote, which are compact varieties with large flower heads. All varieties of lavender are perennial, bushy shrubs with silver, gray, or green linear leaves and purple, violet, blue, or white spiky flowers.

BLENDING PROFILE

Lavender blends well with many other essential oils, especially florals, such as rose, geranium, and chamomile; citruses, such as bergamot, sweet orange, and grapefruit; and herbals, such as sweet marjoram, clary sage, and basil.

TRADITIONAL USES

Dried lavender flowers were traditionally sewn into bags of fine gauze and used to keep clothes fragrant, fresh, and insect free. Lavender water was often used as a simple *eau de toilette*. Lavender essential oil has a long tradition of use in the cosmetics industry, in soaps, talcum powders, and many other products.

THERAPEUTIC PROPERTIES

Analgesic, antidepressant, antiphlogistic, antiseptic, antiviral, bactericide, carminative, cholagogue, cicatrisant,

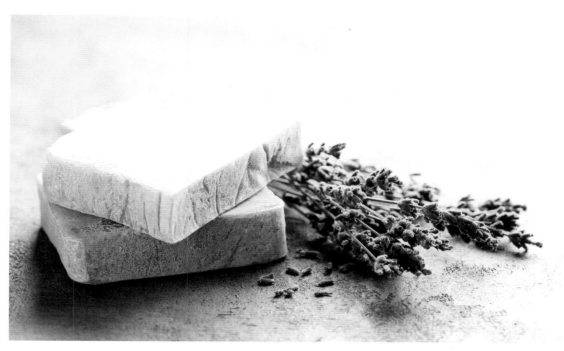

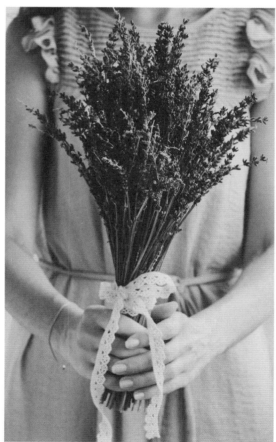

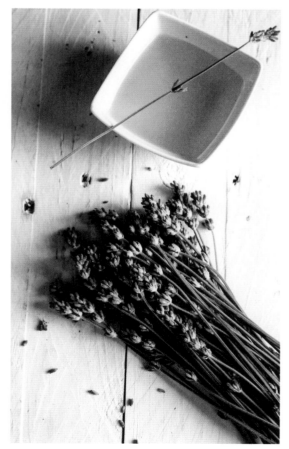

cytophylactic, decongestant, deodorant, emmenagogue, fungicide, hypotensive, nervine, restorative, sedative, sudorific, tonic, and vulnerary. *(See glossary on page 158.)*

Lavender is the most popular, versatile, and widely used of all essential oils in aromatherapy. At first, it almost sounds too good to be true: A cure-all with a reputation lasting thousands of years. However, many of lavender's properties are owing to its principal actions of balancing and normalizing body functions and emotions.

Relaxation and health
Lavender is used particularly in massage, but also in aromatic baths, for muscular aches and pains, insomnia, and to bring about calm and relaxation. Lavender is also valuable in treating colds and flu; not only does it counteract the viruses causing the infection, but it also relieves many of the symptoms. In the case of flu or other feverish conditions, massage is contraindicated, so lavender is best used in steam inhalations and baths.

A cold compress of lavender relieves headaches and migraines. Lavender repels insects, and a drop rubbed over insect bites will lessen the painful sting. Lavender heals minor burns, and is also good for washing and healing minor cuts and grazes when the oil is diluted in a water wash. Alternatively, lavender water, also known as lavender hydrosol, can be used.

Skincare
In skincare, lavender's fresh, delicate, floral fragrance is comfortingly familiar when mixed into skin products such as moisturizing creams and skin toners. Lavender is best suited to normal skin, and it helps to lessen inflammation and acne.

Cosmetic and psychospiritual
Psychologically, lavender is soothing, balancing, and calming, helping with mood swings, depression, and PMS. Its calming, relaxing effects can be used to facilitate meditation. Lavender's balancing qualities can restore harmony to the aura and help to balance the chakras. Lavender is especially associated with the crown chakra and its chakra healing qualities are enhanced if used with an amethyst crystal.

Making a lavender bag

You will need:

- bunch of dried lavender sprigs
- 5–6 in (12–15 cm) square fine gauze or muslin
- needle and thread
- ribbon
- 3 drops lavender essential oil

1. Harvest several sprigs of lavender by cutting off the stalks close to the base of the plant. Tie in a bundle and hang upside down in a cool, dark place for 2 weeks to dry.

2. Spread a sheet of paper or cloth on a table and rub off the dried flowers onto the surface.

3. Place the dried flower heads into the center of the gauze or muslin and fold over. Sew up the edges to create a sealed bag and sew the ribbon into a loop for hanging.

4. Sprinkle the lavender essential oil onto the bag to enhance the fragrance. Hang in a wardrobe or place in a drawer to keep your clothes smelling fresh and fragrant.

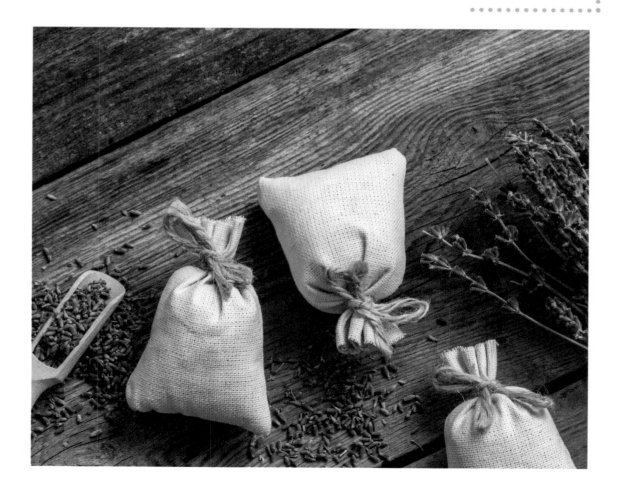

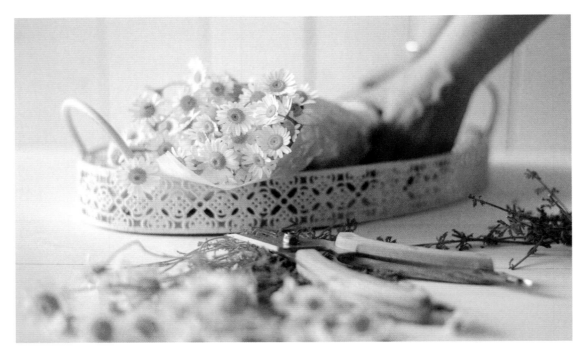

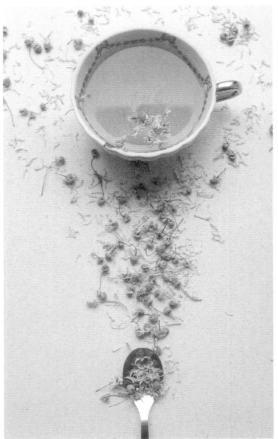

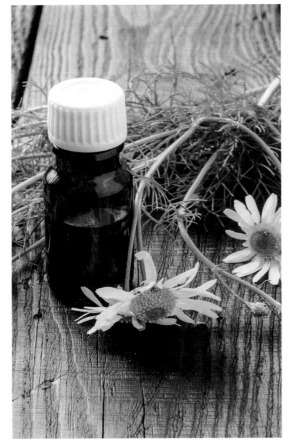

ROMAN CHAMOMILE & GERMAN CHAMOMILE

Anthemis nobilis, Chamaemelum nobile, Matricaria recutita

Botanical Family:
Compositae or Asteraceae

Since antiquity, infused chamomile has been used to alleviate digestive upsets, rashes, insomnia, and headaches.

METHOD OF EXTRACTION:
Roman chamomile is steam distilled from the flowering tops; German chamomile from the dried flower heads.

REGIONS OF ORIGIN:
Australia, Belgium, Bulgaria, England, France, Hungary, Italy, North America, Spain.

CHARACTERISTICS:
Roman chamomile is a clear or pale blue thin oil that easily drops from the bottle dropper. German chamomile is a viscous, deep inky blue.

FRAGRANCE DESCRIPTION:
Roman chamomile has flowery, apple, grassy top notes and bitter, herbaceous undertones. German chamomile has green herbal top notes, with almost fruity, warm, bitter undertones.

SAFE USAGE: Avoid in the first three months of pregnancy.

PLANT DESCRIPTION

Roman chamomile is a perennial herb with a creeping habit, delicate feathery leaves, and daisy-like white flowers. When planted en masse it forms a chamomile lawn—these were popular before plain grass lawns came into fashion. German chamomile is a strongly aromatic annual herb, growing up to 2 feet tall, with delicate feathery leaves and simple, delicate, daisy-like white and yellow flowers.

BLENDING PROFILE

Roman chamomile blends well with most floral and herbal oils, also bergamot, sweet orange, mandarin, frankincense, and patchouli. German chamomile, in small amounts, blends well with most floral, citrus, and herbal oils, also patchouli, frankincense, petitgrain, and benzoin.

TRADITIONAL USES

German chamomile is also called scented mayweed. Chamomile flowers have over 2,000 years of use in the herbal tradition, mainly in Europe. The ancient Egyptians and Moors also used chamomile and, called *maythen*, it is one of the Saxon's nine sacred herbs.

THERAPEUTIC PROPERTIES

Analgesic, anti-allergenic, anti-inflammatory, antiphlogistic, antiseptic, antispasmodic, antiviral, carminative, cholagogue, cicatrisant, digestive, diuretic, emmenagogue, febrifuge, hepatic, nervine, sedative, stomachic, sudorific, and vulnerary. *(See glossary on page 158.)*

Pain relief

Roman chamomile's analgesic properties overlap with those of German chamomile and lavender. A useful tip is to choose lavender for sharp, piercing, sudden pain; German chamomile for hot, red pain, and Roman chamomile for dull, persistent pain.

Roman chamomile is good for alleviating many common ailments in children, particularly teething, and is both gentle and effective. German chamomile is first choice for treating inflammation. It is also excellent for skincare, as is Roman chamomile, but the presence of chamazulene—which gives German chamomile its deep inky blue color—makes it an even more powerful anti-inflammatory. Overall, chamomile is calming, soothing, and comforting.

A good choice for menstrual conditions, chamomile soothes PMT, relieves menstrual cramps, and calms the mood swings and weepiness associated with the menstrual cycle. Chamomile tea helps relieve nausea in pregnancy, as well as general nausea. Chamomile is valuable in treating cystitis. Hot compresses over the abdomen relieve the burning symptoms and allay the anxiety and exhaustion that accompany cystitis (drinking chamomile tea also helps).

Good for hayfever and migraine

Chamomile is useful for hayfever symptoms and can be inhaled from a tissue for quick relief. Alongside drinking chamomile tea, gentle massage with chamomile helps colic, dyspepsia, diarrhea, and indigestion.

Chamomile alleviates headache and migraine when applied to the forehead in a cold compress. Skin allergies, such as eczema, respond well to chamomile mixed into base cream or lotion. Chamomile is good in skincare, having a strong affinity for people with fair complexions, and it helps sensitive, red, and dry skin. Roman chamomile is often used in massage oils, as it promotes relaxation, reduces muscular tension and pain and relieves nervous tension, anxiety, stress, and insomnia.

Calming and restorative

Psychologically, chamomile is calming, balancing, restorative and relaxing. Roman chamomile has an affinity with the throat chakra.

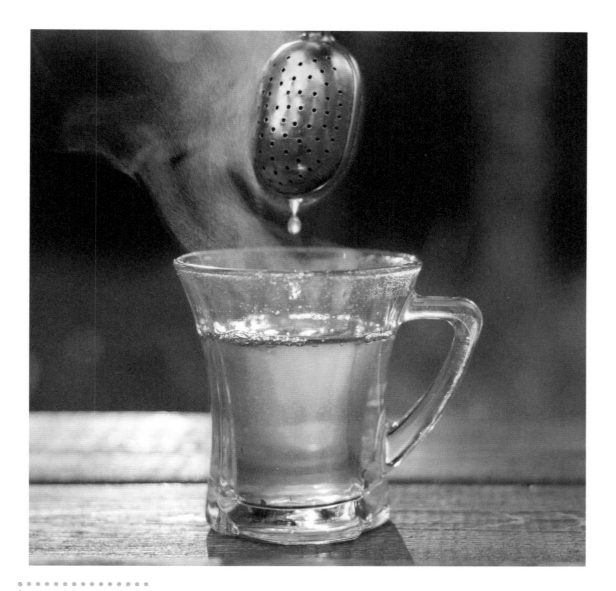

Tummy-calming tea

Overeating, or eating too much rich food, can be relieved by drinking chamomile tea, or "tisane" as herbal teas are also called.

You will need:

- 1 chamomile tea bag or handful of fresh or dried chamomile flowers (preferably organic)

1. Steep the tea bag or flowers in boiling water for 5–10 minutes (strain, if using flowers) and sip slowly. Add a little honey if you don't like the slightly bitter taste.

GERANIUM

Pelargonium graveolens

Botanical Family:
Geraniaceae

The versatility of geranium comes from its cooling and balancing properties. It is highly recommended for menstrual problems, helping to regulate hormones and moods.

METHOD OF EXTRACTION:
Geranium essential oil is steam or water distilled from the flowers, leaves, and stalks.

REGIONS OF ORIGIN:
Réunion and occasionally Central America, China, Congo, Egypt, France, Italy, Japan, Morocco, Russia, South Africa, Spain.

CHARACTERISTICS:
Green or olive green, thin to viscous essential oil that easily drops from the bottle dropper.

FRAGRANCE DESCRIPTION:
Geranium has light, lemon fresh, green herbal top notes and a soft but pronounced rosy, sweet floral undertone. The finest Réunion geranium may have hints of mint and is rosy and sweet fruity.

SAFE USAGE: Avoid in the first three months of pregnancy.

PLANT DESCRIPTION

Geranium is an aromatic, perennial, hairy plant, with serrated leaves. The flowers vary from light pink through to magenta, red, or deep rose. It is also known as stork's bill and by its botanical name, *Pelargonium*. This distinguishes it from the garden perennial cranesbill, also confusingly known as geranium. There are around 700 varieties of geranium, which are mainly used as garden plants, but *graveolens* is the main one cultivated for essential oil. The finest geranium essential oil comes from Réunion and is known as geranium bourbon or rose geranium.

BLENDING PROFILE

Geranium blends well with many other essential oils, but especially bergamot, lavender, basil, rosemary, black pepper, rose, neroli, sandalwood, juniper berry, lemon, patchouli, jasmine, mandarin, and sweet orange.

TRADITIONAL USES

Dioscorides first mentions geranium in his *Materia Medica* and the plant is believed to have originated in South Africa. Geranium was brought to Britain in the 18th century and essential oil distillation began in the Grasse region of France in the 19th century. Geranium has been used historically in the treatment of diarrhea and dysentery. Geranium essential oil has also always been widely used in cosmetics and pharmaceuticals.

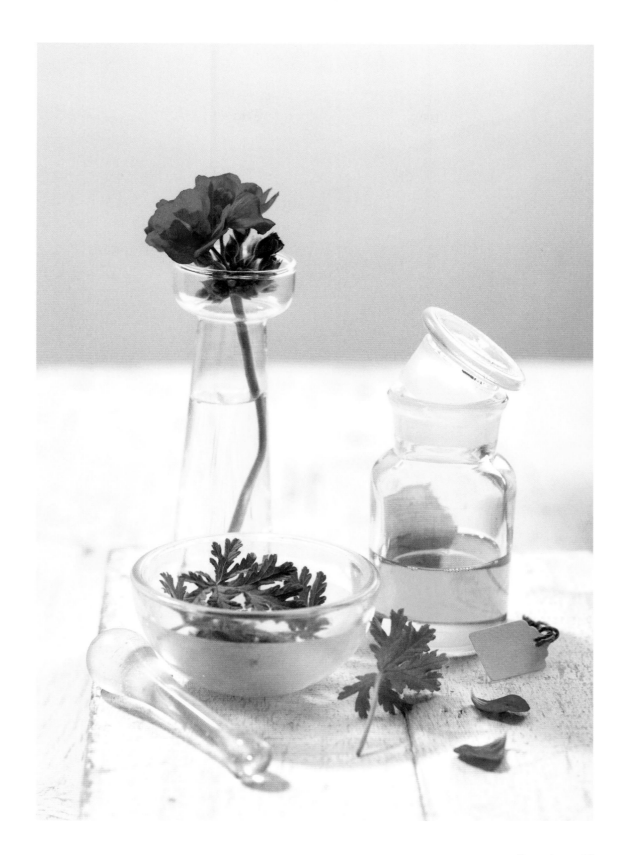

THERAPEUTIC PROPERTIES

Antidepressant, astringent, antiseptic, cicatrisant, cytophylactic, deodorant, diuretic, hemostatic, tonic, vermifuge, and vulnerary. *(See glossary on page 158.)*

Balancing and detoxifying

Geranium is a great balancer owing to its being an adrenal cortex stimulant, and it helps to regulate hormones and moods. One of the most useful essential oils to detoxify the lymphatic system and help eliminate cellulite, geranium is often included in lymphatic drainage massage blends, together with rosemary, citrus and spice oils and juniper berry, to treat fluid retention and edema of the lower legs.

Geranium heals wounds and burns quickly owing to its hemostatic properties, and also lessens bruising. It makes a good deodorant, and can be used to freshen rooms, particularly when blended with bergamot and cypress. Overall, geranium is balancing, uplifting, and refreshing.

Fragrant and uplifting

Because geranium smells a little like rose—but is cheaper—it is used in the perfume industry to give a rose-like scent and to "extend" or adulterate rose. Geranium is a valuable skincare essential oil, and it is helpful in balancing sebum production. Geranium is especially good for menstrual problems, as it balances the hormones. This, combined with its antidepressant, uplifting qualities, means geranium might be helpful in massage blends for women who have difficulty becoming pregnant. It is also useful to help relieve symptoms of the menopause.

Geranium helps regulate the nervous system and its action is both sedative and uplifting. Psychologically, it creates a sense of security and comfort, and is gently elevating and balancing. Geranium is reputed to strengthen the flow of subtle energy, or *chi*, and is valuable in treating anxiety associated with nervous debility. Geranium is useful in perfumes to bring about a balanced harmony, and to counteract excessive mood swings.

Geranium spray deodorant

Geranium's antibacterial properties and delicate fragrance make it an effective, natural deodorant.

You will need:

- 1 x 3½ fl oz (100 ml) dark glass spray bottle
- 1 tsp perfumer's alcohol (see page 40)
- 20 drops geranium essential oil
- 15 drops bergamot essential oil
- 10 drops cypress essential oil
- flower water, such as rose water, to top up

1. Measure the perfumer's alcohol into the bottle and add the essential oils. Shake well to dissolve.

2. Top up with flower water, allowing enough space to accommodate the spray pump.

3. Shake well to mix the ingredients.

4. Label the bottle with the ingredients, amounts used, and the date. Use as an underarm deodorant when required.

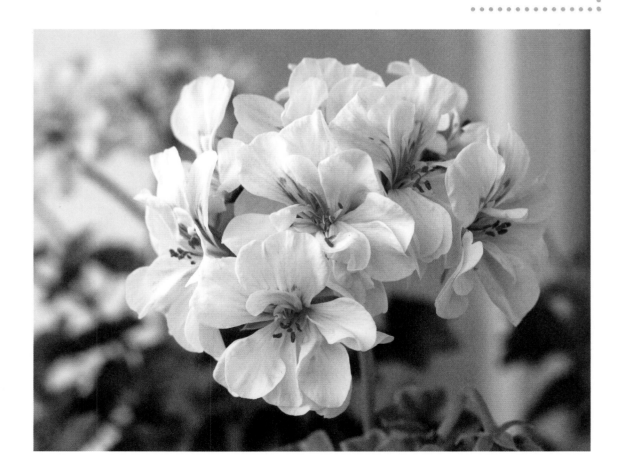

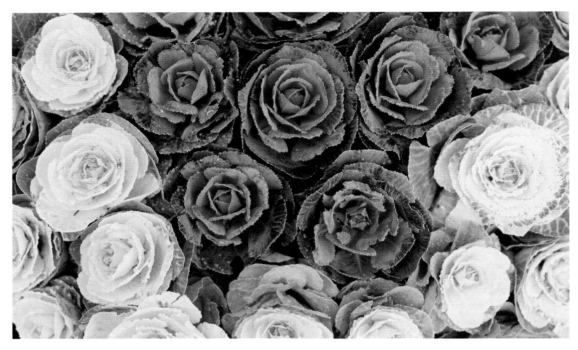

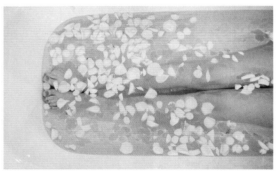

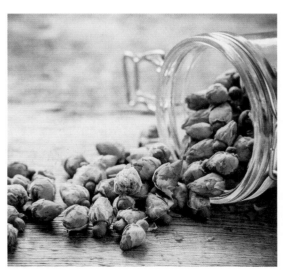

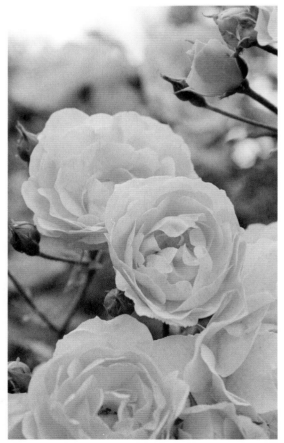

ROSE DAMASK—ROSE OTTO & ROSE CABBAGE—ROSE ABSOLUTE

Rosa damascena, Rosa centifolia

Botanical Family:
Rosaceae

Rose has often been described as the "queen of flowers," and for many aromatherapists there is no finer essential oil.

METHOD OF EXTRACTION:
The essential oil (rose otto or attar) is steam distilled from the petals and whole flowers of rose damask. Rose absolute, or rose maroc, is produced from rosa centifolia by solvent extraction from the petals.

REGIONS OF ORIGIN:
Bulgaria, China, France, Italy, Morocco, Turkey.

CHARACTERISTICS:
Rose essential oil is pale or green yellow. It can be solid but a little warmth turns it liquid. Rose absolute is viscous and varies from browny red to greeny orange.

FRAGRANCE DESCRIPTION:
Rose has deep, sweet, floral top notes with dusky, honeyed, rosy undertones.

SAFE USAGE: Avoid in the first three months of pregnancy.

PLANT DESCRIPTION

Rose damask produces pink or red flowers in late spring and early summer. It is known as Bulgarian or Turkish rose. *Rosa centifolia* or rose cabbage produces pink flowers in late spring and early summer.

BLENDING PROFILE

Rose blends well with other floral oils, also bergamot, lemon, clary sage, sandalwood, melissa, frankincense, palmarosa, patchouli, myrrh, and benzoin.

TRADITIONAL USES

Ancient Romans used rose flowers and rose water at feasts, weddings, and funerals. Culpepper used rose in ancient English medicine as an anti-inflammatory. Rose petals and buds are a main ingredient in pot pourri. Rose oil is used extensively in the cosmetics industry, although the high cost of true rose means much adulterated and synthetic rose is substituted. Rose water, a by-product of steam distillation, is used in Middle Eastern cuisine and in many countries for its skincare properties.

THERAPEUTIC PROPERTIES

Antidepressant, antiphlogistic, antiseptic, antispasmodic, antiviral, aphrodisiac, astringent, bactericidal, choleretic, cicatrisant, depurative, emmenagogue, hemostatic, hepatic, laxative, nervine, sedative, tonic, and uterine. *(See glossary on page 158.)*

Emotionally healing

Rose absolute is cheaper than rose otto, but the wonderful healing and skincare properties of either rose are definitely worth using. Rose otto and absolute both smell gorgeous, although they differ slightly. Rose is quite safe to use if you follow the guidelines and, as the aroma is strong and tenacious, 1–2% dilution is sufficient.

Rose comforts the heart in grief, helping the bereaved, as well as those grieving for a finished relationship. Rose is a tonic of the physical heart and it also lifts the spirits, allays anxiety, fear and anger, and is nurturing. Overall, rose is tender, uplifting, and soothing.

Beneficial for women

Rose is first choice in treating female reproductive problems, helping alleviate PMS and menopausal symptoms, and regulating periods; it may even help women who have problems conceiving. It has a tonic, purifying effect on the uterus and helps those suffering from postnatal depression and after suffering a miscarriage. The aphrodisiac qualities of rose help women express femininity and sexuality by alleviating anxiety and nervous tension, and inspiring a confident sensuality. Rose is best used in massage oil or perfume where its wonderful fragrance is most appreciated.

Excellent in skincare

Rose is emollient and hydrating, which together with its delicious fragrance, make it valuable in skincare. Mixed into lotions, creams, and face oils, rose treats mature, dry, inflamed, and sensitive skins but is useful for all skin types. It has a tonic and astringent effect on the fine capillaries in the face and lessens redness. Rose makes a special addition to massage and bath oils, and is extensively used in perfumes.

Psychologically, rose alleviates sadness and disappointment. It relieves anxiety and grief and strengthens the inner spirit. Rose is associated with the heart chakra, opening and healing the heart to love. Energetically, rose is classified as cool and moist so it is indicated for hot, red, inflamed conditions.

Rose facial oil

This simple rose face oil may be costly but it is very effective and lovely to use.

You will need:

- 1 x 1 fl oz (30 ml) dark glass bottle
- 4 tsp apricot kernel oil
- 2 tsp rosehip seed oil
- 6 drops rose otto or absolute

1. Mix the apricot, rosehip, and rose together thoroughly and pour into the bottle.

2. Label with the ingredients, amounts, and date. Use a few drops every morning and night either before, or instead of, your usual moisturizer.

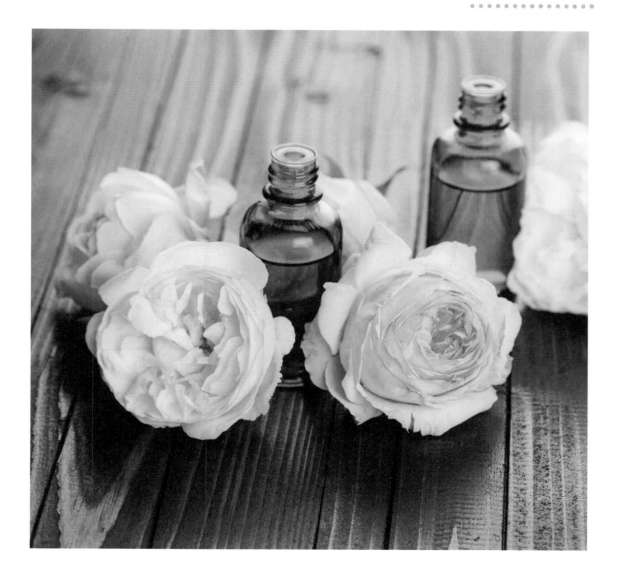

NEROLI

Citrus aurantium

*Botanical Family:
Rutaceae*

Neroli has long been considered the best choice to treat acute anxiety. It can help alleviate panic attacks, hysteria, and shock, as well as helping all chronic emotional nervous conditions.

METHOD OF EXTRACTION:
The essential oil is steam distilled from the flowers of neroli bigarade. It can be confused with neroli Portugal or citronier. An orange flower absolute is also available: It is expensive and may be adulterated with synthetics.

REGIONS OF ORIGIN:
Algeria, Egypt, France, Italy, Morocco, Tunisia.

CHARACTERISTICS:
Neroli is a pale yellow, thin essential oil that easily drops from the bottle dropper. It is also called orange flower blossom or orange blossom.

FRAGRANCE DESCRIPTION:
Neroli has delicate, fresh, floral top notes with heady, bittersweet undertones.

SAFE USAGE: Neroli is a safe essential oil with no contraindications.

PLANT DESCRIPTION

The bitter orange is an evergreen tree with a smooth gray trunk, dark green leaves, small fruit, and fragrant white flowers. As well as neroli from the flowers, the tree also produces petitgrain essential oil from the leaves (and sometimes twigs), and bitter orange from the fruit.

BLENDING PROFILE

Neroli blends well with almost all essential oils, but especially lavender, melissa, rose, jasmine, frankincense, sandalwood, clary sage, and bergamot.

TRADITIONAL USES

The oil is named after the 17th-century Italian Princess of Nerola, who loved it and used it extensively. The flowers and oil were traditionally used for all nervous conditions, especially when these manifested as gastrointestinal complaints, and also for insomnia. Traditionally used in wedding bouquets, neroli calms and soothes the nerves before major events. Orange flower water, a by-product of steam distillation of the flowers, is used throughout the Middle East in cooking and skincare.

THERAPEUTIC PROPERTIES

Antidepressant, antiseptic, antispasmodic, aphrodisiac, bactericidal, carminative, cicatrisant, cordial, deodorant, digestive, sedative, and tonic. *(See glossary on page 158.)*

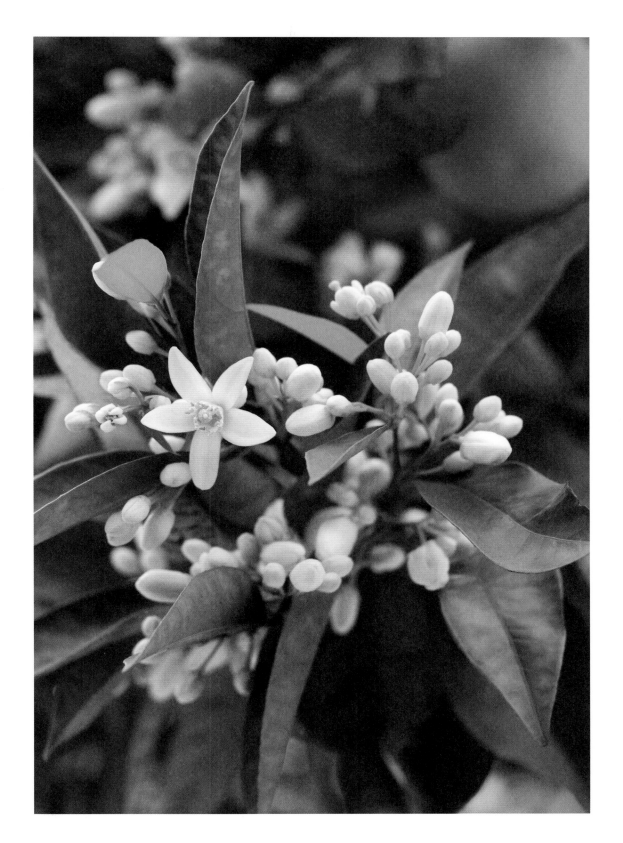

Rejuvenates mature skin

Valuable in skincare, neroli helps the regeneration of healthy new skin cells and rejuvenates mature skin. Neroli is good for all skin types, but especially valuable for mature, dry, and sensitive skins. The beautiful fragrance of this essential oil makes it a wonderful addition to all skincare products, as well as perfumes, and massage and bath oils.

Relieves anxiety

Neroli is useful for treating diarrhea. Its antispasmodic properties relieve spasm in the smooth muscles of the intestines, while its calming effect relieves the anxiety or shock that can cause or aggravate diarrhea. A few drops of neroli in a bath or on the pillow can relieve insomnia. A gentle and subtle aphrodisiac, neroli is useful for those who are nervous of sexual encounters. Brides traditionally held a bouquet of orange flower blossom, which they could smell to calm their nerves and give them confidence.

Emotionally calming

Psychologically, neroli is calming and uplifting, especially for those who are easily agitated, emotionally unstable, or insecure, and it eases the intensity of strong emotions. Neroli is associated with innocence and purity, and inspires creativity. It is a useful aid to meditation and facilitates spiritual healing.

Neroli soothes problems of an urgent emotional or psychological origin and it also helps those with long-term, chronic anxiety. Overall, neroli is calming, soothing, and uplifting and is gentle enough to use in small amounts with children. Neroli has an affinity with the heart and helps relieve hypertension by having a regulating effect on heart rhythm and soothing nervous palpitations.

Neroli flower spray

Neroli is effective at relieving nervous conditions and is especially associated with bridal bouquets. Wedding guests can benefit from the stress and anxiety-relieving properties of neroli in a similar way by making and wearing this simple corsage or buttonhole flower spray.

You will need:

- a few artificial (silk) white flower sprays (orange flower blossom, if possible)
- florist's wire
- 2–3 drops neroli essential oil
- safety pin

1. Create an arrangement with the flower sprays.

2. Twist the florist's wire around the stalks, near the base, to hold everything firmly in place. Use the safety pin to go round the whole spray and, if possible, conceal the wire.

3. Carefully drip the neroli onto the flowers and then pin the corsage onto a jacket, blouse, or dress.

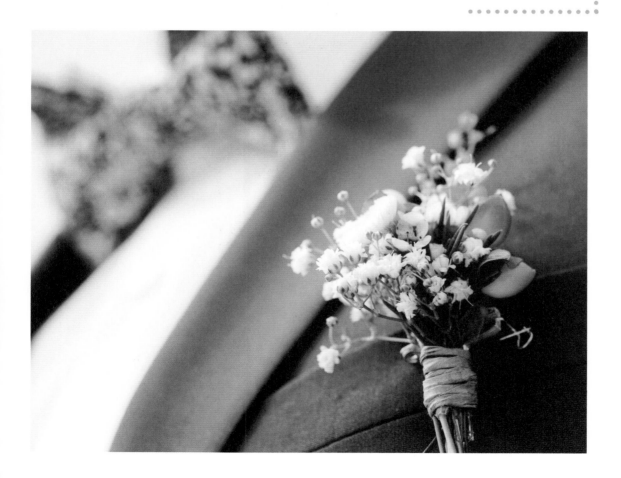

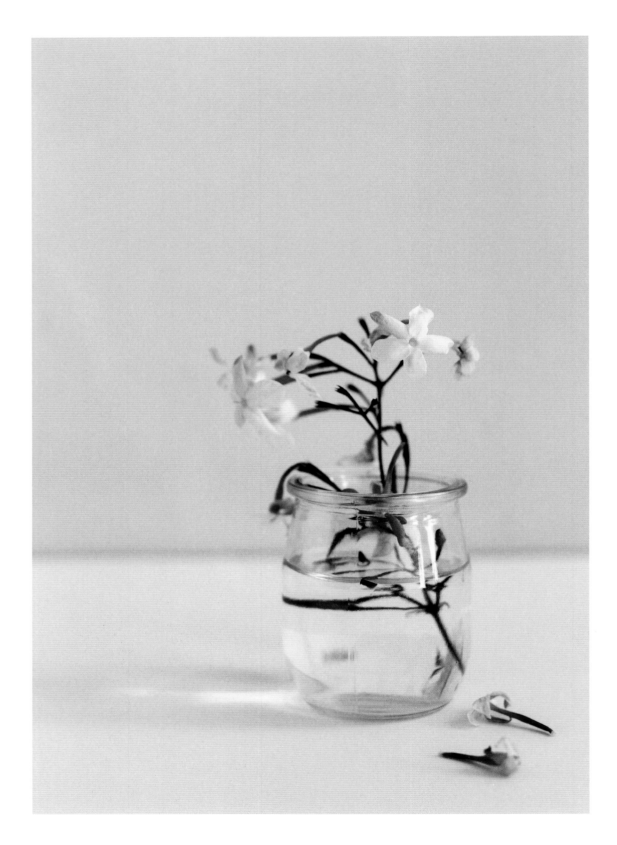

JASMINE

Jasminum grandiflorum

Botanical Family:
Oleaceae

The powerful floral fragrance of jasmine is emotionally warming and uplifting, making jasmine the best essential oil to inspire confidence.

METHOD OF EXTRACTION:
Jasmine absolute is produced by solvent extraction from the flowers.

REGIONS OF ORIGIN:
Algeria, China, Egypt, France, India, Italy, Morocco.

CHARACTERISTICS:
Jasmine is a dark orange-brown, viscous absolute that easily drops from the bottle dropper.

FRAGRANCE DESCRIPTION:
Jasmine has a powerful, heady fragrance. This can be overwhelming, but once diluted, it becomes softer and more subtle. Jasmine has sweet, floral, exotic top notes, and heady, warm, honeyed undertones.

SAFE USAGE: Avoid in the first three months of pregnancy, especially if there is a history of miscarriage. Use in small amounts only.

PLANT DESCRIPTION

Jasmine is a perennial, fast-growing, climbing shrub, with fine, small green or variegated leaves and delicate flowers—usually white, but may also be pink or yellow. In addition to *grandiflorum*, there are two other species; *auriculatum* and *sambac*. Jasmine *sambac* comes from India, where it is called mogra. Jasmine *sambac* absolute is also used in aromatherapy and has a more intense, wild, and untamed fragrance than *grandiflorum*.

BLENDING PROFILE

Jasmine blends well with the citrus oils, also clary sage, rose, sandalwood, rosewood, frankincense, neroli, cypress, ginger, cardamom, Roman chamomile, and melissa.

TRADITIONAL USES

Jasmine flowers have been used since ancient times for religious ceremonies and adornment. From the 15th century, jasmine was cultivated in India, Afghanistan, China, Iran, and Nepal. It was introduced to Europe around 1600, having been brought to Spain by the Moors. In China jasmine flowers of *grandiflorum* were used to treat liver conditions and dysentery, while jasmine *sambac* was used to treat conjunctivitis, ulcers, and tumors. Jasmine has also been used as an aphrodisiac and to assist in childbirth.

THERAPEUTIC PROPERTIES

Analgesic, antidepressant, anti-inflammatory, antiseptic, antispasmodic, aphrodisiac, galactagogue, parturient, nervine, sedative, tonic, and uterine. *(See glossary on page 158.)*

Liberating and sensual

Jasmine helps us to liberate our inhibitions. It is a powerful antidepressant of a stimulating nature and these qualities combine to help those suffering from lack of confidence, vacillation, indecision and the lethargy born of depression. Perfumes and massage oils are the best methods to make the most of the delicious but costly fragrance. Overall, jasmine is intoxicating, euphoric, and aphrodisiac.

In a similar way to rose, jasmine is useful in treating the female reproductive system. It is excellent for use during childbirth: When massaged over the lower back and abdomen in the early stages of labor, it works to alleviate pain and strengthen contractions. Later on, it can also help to expel the placenta. Jasmine also strengthens the male sexual organs and can be used to help treat enlargement of the prostrate gland. Unsurprisingly, jasmine is also one of the most powerful aphrodisiacs available in the aromatherapist's collection, and can help couples reignite their sexual spark.

Euphoric fragrance

The lovely fragrance of jasmine makes it useful in skincare, especially for hot, dry, sensitive, inflamed, and mature skins. A single drop blended with other essential oils can make any skin cream smell wonderful. It is best used in small amounts—1 drop or 1% dilution is ideal, as the fragrance can be overwhelming and may even cause headaches if too much is used.

Jasmine is effective in treating nervous anxiety, restlessness, and depression. Psychologically, jasmine inspires euphoria, helping to restore confidence and optimism. Jasmine warms and opens the emotions, helping those who are habitually repressed and shy. It is associated with intuitive wisdom, and is useful for insight meditation. Jasmine releases inhibitions, liberates the imagination, and inspires creativity.

Sensual massage oil

This sensuous blend can reinvigorate a bored, tired sex life. All the oils (except bergamot, which adds a light fresh note to the blend), have aphrodisiac properties.

You will need:

- 1 x 1 fl oz (20 ml) dark glass bottle
- 4 tsp sweet almond oil
- 2 drops jasmine absolute (grandiflorum or sambac)
- 3 drops bergamot essential oil
- 1 drop clary sage essential oil
- 1 drop black pepper essential oil
- 1 drop patchouli essential oil

1. Measure the sweet almond oil into the bottle.

2. Carefully drip the correct number of drops of each essential oil into the bottle. Don't be tempted to add extra drops, as you might create a smell that is too strong and overpowering—definitely not sensual! Shake gently to mix the oils.

3. Label the bottle with the ingredients, amounts used, and the date. Create an erotic atmosphere in a suitable place and begin giving your partner a massage with the oil, then see where this fragrant adventure leads you.

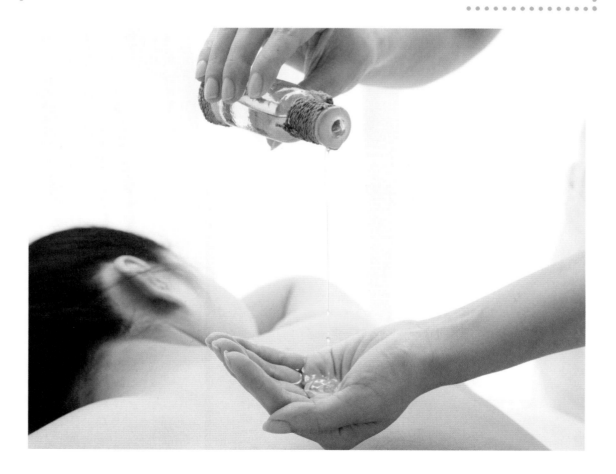

YLANG YLANG

Cananga odorata

*Botanical Family:
Annonaceae*

Ylang ylang means "flower of flowers" in Malayan, and it is much used in the perfume industry for its voluptuous, exotic fragrance.

METHOD OF EXTRACTION:
The essential oil is steam and water distilled from the flowers. Ylang ylang extra has the best fragrance and most active therapeutic qualities. Ylang ylang complete is distilled traditionally and is a premium natural essential oil.

REGIONS OF ORIGIN:
Comoros Islands, Indonesia, Madagascar, Philippines, Réunion.

CHARACTERISTICS:
Ylang ylang is a pale yellow, viscous oil that easily drops from the bottle dropper.

FRAGRANCE DESCRIPTION:
Ylang ylang extra has intensely sweet, fruity, floral, creamy tropical top notes, and woody, balsamic undertones. Ylang ylang complete has warm, almond undertones with hints of spice and sweet, narcotic floral top notes.

PLANT DESCRIPTION

The cananga tree is a tall evergreen with branches that bend down. It produces many large yellow and white flowers year round, with an intensely powerful scent.

BLENDING PROFILE

Ylang ylang blends well with most floral, spice, and citrus oils, also rosewood, patchouli, vetivert, petitgrain, and sandalwood.

TRADITIONAL USES

In Java, Indonesia, the flowers are scattered on bridal beds, reflecting ylang ylang's aphrodisiac properties. They can also be macerated in olive oil and used over the whole body to protect skin and hair from the sun. In Victorian England, ylang ylang was the main ingredient of Macassar, a popular male hair application. Ylang ylang is much used in the cosmetics industry, particularly in soap, as the fragrance is so tenacious.

THERAPEUTIC PROPERTIES

Antidepressant, antiseptic, aphrodisiac, astringent, hypotensive, and sedative. *(See glossary on page 158.)*

Soothing and erotic

An important use of ylang ylang in aromatherapy is in helping reduce high blood pressure, especially when accompanied by heart palpitations. Ylang ylang also

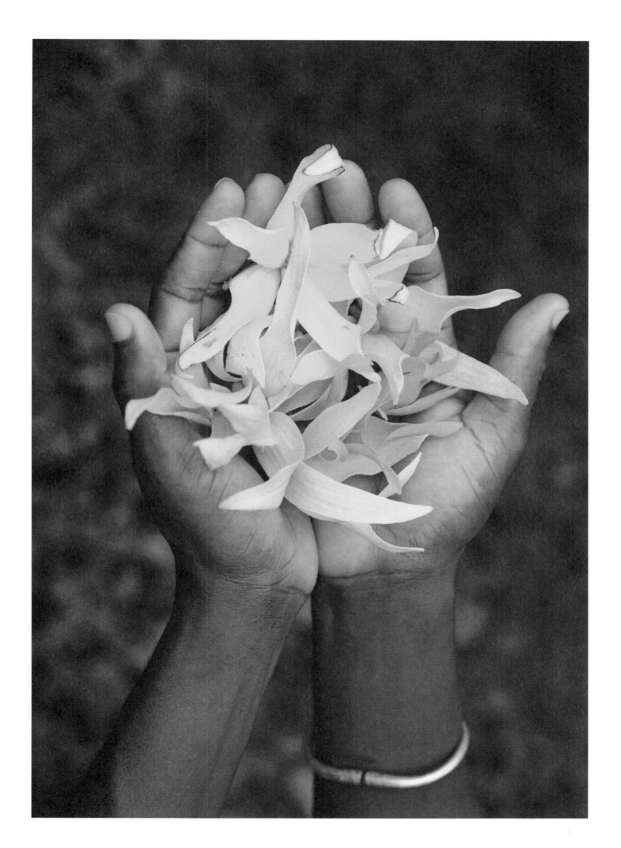

treats anxiety, anger, shock, and fear. It helps to slow over-rapid breathing, and reduces "fight or flight" syndrome. Overall, ylang ylang is soothing, erotic, and euphoric.

Balancing and moisturizing

In skincare ylang ylang is valued for its sweet, pleasing fragrance. It is especially suited to oily skin, although its balancing action on sebum production makes it useful for all skin types. Traditionally, the flowers are macerated in coconut oil—a product called Monoi de Tahiti—and used as a hairdressing product. Monoi de Tahiti is also often incorporated into body butters, and skin and hand creams for its moisturizing properties and lovely fragrance.

Use only small amounts of ylang ylang and not for long periods of time. The perfume can become sickly and heavy and might cause headaches and nausea. Blending it with lemon, bergamot, and other fresh-smelling essential oils lightens the fragrance. Ylang ylang also blends well with spice oils, which help alleviate the cloying sweetness.

Relaxing and anti-depressant

Ylang ylang can help treat frigidity and impotence, particularly when used in blends for full body massage, which helps "reunite" the whole physical body with mind, emotions, and spirit. In perfume, its sweet, voluptuous, and erotic fragrance can help release inhibitions and bring out fiery passion. Ylang ylang is particularly suited to women, and can help them find their inner femininity, confidence, and sensuality.

Adding ylang ylang to your bath promotes relaxation and aids sleep. It is valuable in treating depression, especially when the depression is accompanied by a lot of nervous tension. Ylang ylang is one of the most helpful essential oils to use with meditation to counteract anger. Psychologically, ylang ylang calms, uplifts, creates a sense of peace, and aids self-expression of repressed inner feelings.

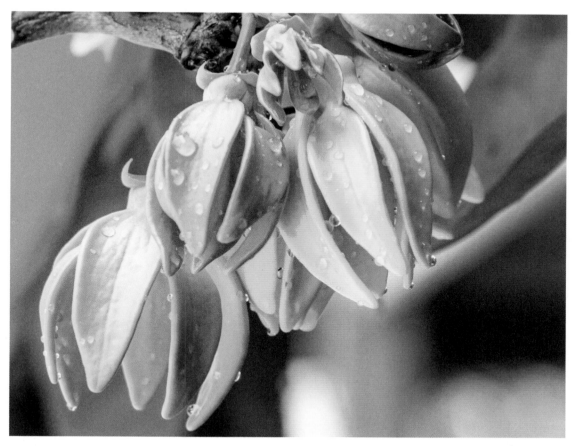

Ylang ylang scalp tonic

Adding ylang ylang to base shampoo makes a sweet-smelling hair product that has a stimulating effect on the scalp, promoting hair growth. Available from health stores, base shampoo is made from natural ingredients with no added color or perfume, and used as a base for your own blends.

You will need:

- 1 x 7 fl oz (200 ml) bottle of base shampoo
- 40 drops ylang ylang essential oil

1. Pour the shampoo into a jug and gently but thoroughly stir in the drops of ylang ylang, avoiding creating air bubbles.

2. Pour back into the bottle and use as required.

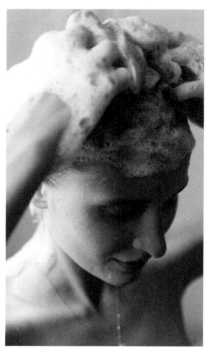

BERGAMOT

Citrus bergamia

*Botanical Family:
Rutaceae*

A key ingredient of eau de Cologne, bergamot is regarded as the finest of the citrus oils. It is an excellent choice to treat depression and anxiety.

METHOD OF EXTRACTION:
Cold pressed. The peel of the nearly ripe bergamot fruit is mechanically squeezed to express the essential oil.

REGIONS OF ORIGIN:
Corsica, Guinea, Italy, Ivory Coast, Morocco.

CHARACTERISTICS:
Bergamot is a pale green, thin essential oil that easily drops from the bottle dropper.

FRAGRANCE DESCRIPTION:
Bergamot has fruity, sweet, lemon, fresh top notes with warm, floral, balsamic undertones.

SAFE USAGE: If you have very sensitive skin use only 1–2 drops. Do not use before sun exposure unless you use bergamot FCF, which has been treated to remove photosensitizing components. Use only 3–4 drops in the bath.

PLANT DESCRIPTION

The bergamot tree was originally only grown in Italy but is now grown more widely. The tree produces small citrus fruits that ripen from green to yellow, but the fruit is too sour to eat.

BLENDING PROFILE

Bergamot blends well with other citrus oils, floral oils, and absolutes. It also blends well with cypress, sandalwood, juniper berry, coriander, black pepper, cardamom, ginger, clary sage, rosemary, sweet marjoram, and frankincense.

TRADITIONAL USES

Bergamot is named after the northern Italian city of Bergamo, where the oil was first traded. A key ingredient of eau de Cologne, bergamot was also used in Italian folk medicine to treat fever and worms. Bergamot production increased in the 16th century when the fragrance became popular. It is still used to flavor Earl Grey tea and is also widely used in the cosmetics industry.

THERAPEUTIC PROPERTIES

Analgesic, antiseptic, antidepressant, antiviral, antispasmodic, carminative, cicatrisant, cordial, deodorant, digestive, febrifuge, sedative, stomachic, tonic, vermifuge, and vulnerary. *(See glossary on page 158.)*

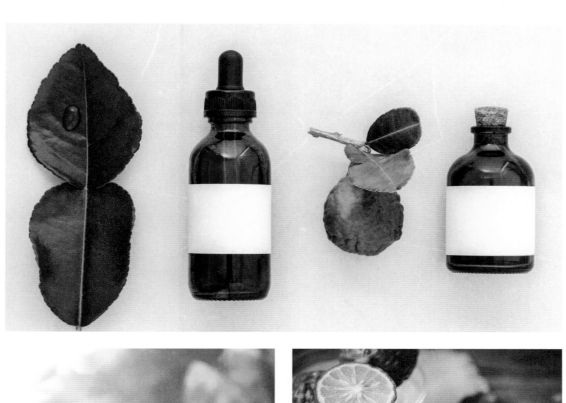

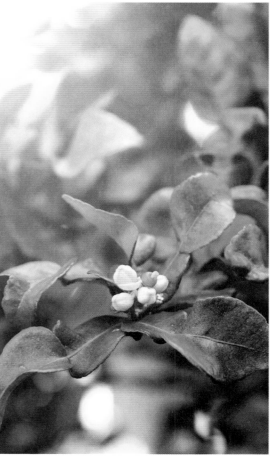

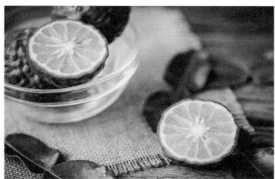

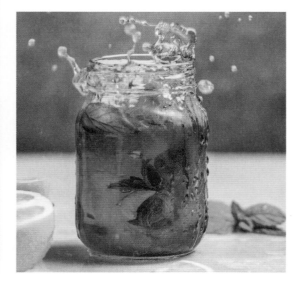

Cheering

Bergamot is used to treat depression and anxiety. It is also first choice for urinary tract infections and cystitis. Chronic sufferers of cystitis often become tense and anxious with the onset of symptoms—a local wash of bergamot both calms the nerves and relieves the symptoms. Overall, bergamot is cheering, uplifting, and calming.

Relieves symptoms of skin conditions

The lovely fragrance and powerful antiseptic qualities of bergamot make it a valuable addition to skincare, and it is especially suited to oily skins (as it is phototoxic, care must be taken on sunny days). Bergamot also helps treat acne, eczema, and psoriasis. Bergamot has been found to inhibit herpes simplex, the virus that causes cold sores. When combined with tea tree or lavender it also treats chicken pox and shingles.

Heartwarming and reviving

Bergamot has a regulating, normalizing effect on the appetite, and is useful in convalescence and for those who are dieting. Bergamot may also be useful to those suffering from anorexia. Used in the bath it is cooling for feverish conditions. Psychologically, bergamot is reviving, soothing, and balancing. Its sunny, antidepressant qualities can help treat Seasonal Affective Disorder, and it is cheering on cold, gray, winter days. Bergamot is heartwarming and has an affinity with the heart chakra, gently relieving sadness, depression, and grief.

Bergamot eau de Cologne

Perfumer's alcohol is widely available and allows you to blend essential oils to produce a clear perfume, although some essential oils may add a little color.

You will need:

- 1 x 1 fl oz (30 ml) dark glass bottle
- 6 tsp perfumer's alcohol
- 14 drops bergamot essential oil
- 10 drops lemon essential oil
- 8 drops sweet orange essential oil
- 6 drops neroli essential oil
- 3 drops lavender essential oil
- 2 drops rosemary essential oil
- 1 drop thyme essential oil
- 1 drop clove essential oil
- 1 drop benzoin essential oil
- 2 drops petitgrain essential oil

1. Half fill the bottle with perfumer's alcohol, then drop in the correct amount of drops of each essential oil. Don't be tempted to make the perfume any stronger by using more essential oils, as this may cause a skin reaction or irritation.

2. Gently shake the bottle for a few minutes to fully mix and dissolve the oils into the perfumer's alcohol.

3. Top up the bottle with perfumer's alcohol, leaving enough space so the ingredients can be fully mixed by a further gentle swishing.

4. Label and date the bottle. Use sparingly—a dab behind the ears and on the insides of the wrists is sufficient for you to enjoy the fragrance.

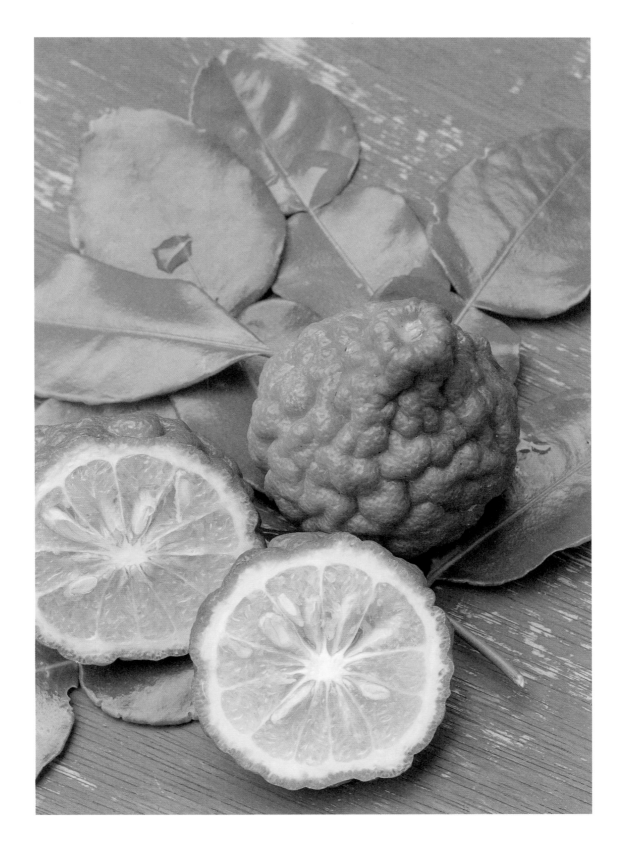

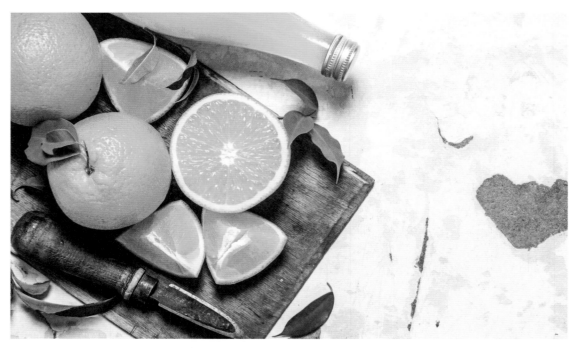

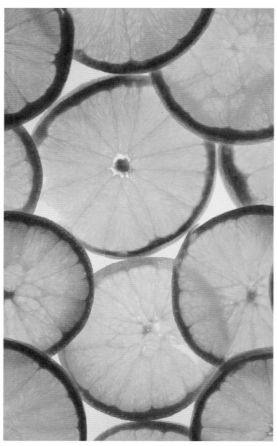

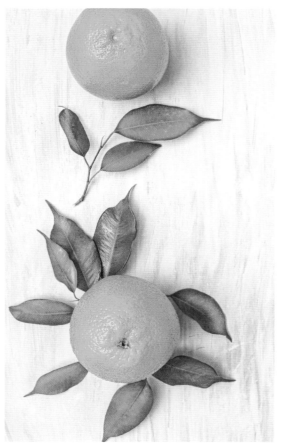

SWEET ORANGE

Citrus sinensis

Botanical Family:
Rutaceae

Sweet orange is familiar, comforting, joyful, and warming.
It is one of the most popular and widely used essential oils.

METHOD OF EXTRACTION:
Cold pressed. The peel of the nearly ripe orange fruit is mechanically squeezed to express the essential oil.

REGIONS OF ORIGIN:
Australia, Brazil, Israel, Italy, North America.

CHARACTERISTICS:
Sweet orange is a yellow to dark orange, thin essential oil that easily drops from the bottle dropper.

FRAGRANCE DESCRIPTION:
Sweet orange has sweet, fresh, fruity top notes with radiant, sensuous undertones. It smells unmistakably of orange!

SAFE USAGE: Sweet orange is one of the safest essential oils and there are no contraindications, although if you have very sensitive skin, use in moderation.

PLANT DESCRIPTION

The sweet orange tree is smaller than the bitter orange, and has dark green, shiny leaves, fragrant white flowers, and abundant fruit. There are many varieties, such as Navel, Valencia, and Jaffa.

BLENDING PROFILE

Sweet orange blends well with the other citrus oils and spice oils, also sandalwood, neroli, clary sage, myrrh, geranium, palmarosa, petitgrain, frankincense, and cypress.

TRADITIONAL USES

Sweet orange trees probably originated in the region between the Himalayas and southwest China and the word orange comes from the Arabic *narandji*. They were introduced to Europe in the 16th century by Portuguese explorers, and then later into the Americas by Columbus. They then spread to the West Indies. In ancient China, dried orange peel was used to treat coughs, colds, and anorexia. Sweet orange essential oil is used these days extensively in the flavoring industry.

THERAPEUTIC PROPERTIES

Antidepressant, antibacterial, antifungal, antiseptic, antispasmodic, carminative, cholagogue, digestive, lymphatic stimulant, sedative, stomachic, and tonic. *(See glossary on page 158.)*

Suitable for children

Sweet orange is gentle enough to use with children, who enjoy its fruity fragrance, and it can be used to aid sleep and relieve tummy upsets in childhood. It is also excellent for settling adult digestive upsets. It has a normalizing, regulating effect on the digestive system that is beneficial for cramps, diarrhea, and flatulence. To help relieve constipation, it is blended with sweet marjoram and black pepper and used in local massage over the abdomen. Overall, sweet orange is tonic, soothing, and refreshing.

Inner radiance

Sweet orange is good in massage and baths for anxiety, stress, and insomnia. It has a mild tonic effect on the lymphatic system. Sweet orange can also be used in skincare, as it is soothing and has mild regenerative properties, which help restore a natural radiance to skin.

Psychologically, sweet orange is cheering and uplifting, helping you find laughter and joy in life. It reduces fear of the unknown and relieves self-doubt, helping you find, or regain, an inner radiance and optimism. Sweet orange helps stimulate stagnant subtle energies and refreshes the spirit and emotions.

Sweet orange bubble bath

This recipe is for children over the age of five who have trouble sleeping. It's fun and creative to involve your child in making the recipe, as they will enjoy using it more.

You will need:

- a squeezy or pump bottle
- 7 fl oz (200 ml) unfragranced base bubble bath or liquid soap
- 20–40 drops sweet orange essential oil
- 1–2 drops orange food coloring

1. Pour the base bubble bath or liquid soap into a jug. For each 3½ fl oz (100 ml) of base bubble bath, drop in 20 drops of sweet orange essential oil. This is 1% dilution, which is a low, safe percentage to use for children.

2. Begin to stir in the drops of essential oil gently with a chopstick or similar. Be careful not to stir vigorously, as this will make the mixture frothy with lots of air bubbles, which you don't want until it goes into the bath.

3. As you stir in the sweet orange, drop in the orange food coloring to build up to the color your child wants (don't put too much in at the beginning).

4. When finished, pour the bubble bath into the bottle. You can make a pretty label, listing the ingredients and saying it was made by you and your child. Pour 1–2 teaspoons under running water for a calming bath.

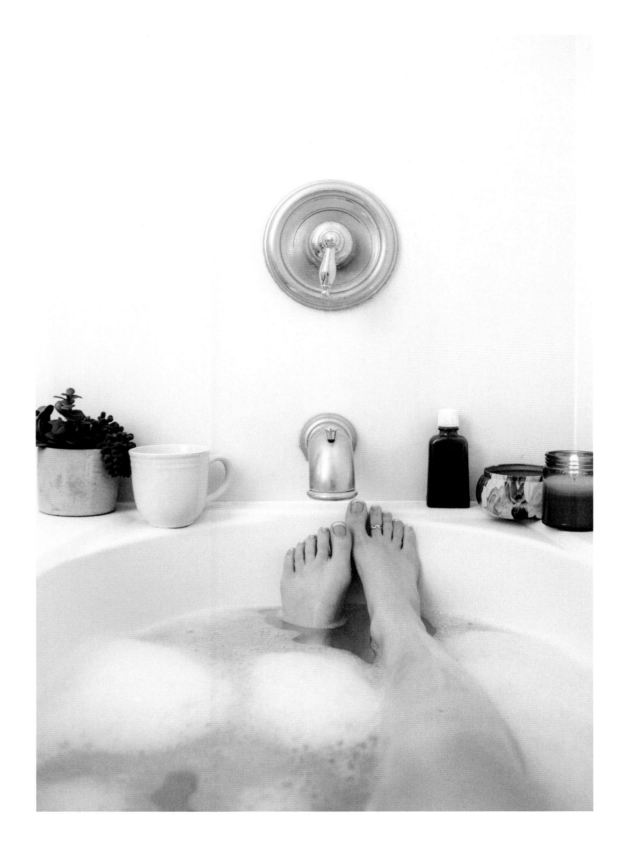

MANDARIN

Citrus reticulata

*Botanical Family:
Rutaceae*

Mandarin is one of the safest essential oils, suitable for all the family. Use it to help switch off an overactive mind and promote restful sleep.

METHOD OF EXTRACTION:
Cold pressed. The peel of the nearly ripe mandarin fruit is mechanically squeezed to express the essential oil.

REGIONS OF ORIGIN:
Algeria, Brazil, China, Cyprus, Greece, Italy, Southeast Asia, Spain.

CHARACTERISTICS:
Mandarin is a yellow-orange, thin essential oil that easily drops from the bottle dropper.

FRAGRANCE DESCRIPTION:
Mandarin has delicate but intense sweet, citrus top notes with deep, warm, fruity—almost floral—undertones.

SAFE USAGE: Mandarin is one of the safest essential oils and there are no contraindications.

PLANT DESCRIPTION

Mandarin is a small evergreen tree with glossy leaves, fragrant flowers, and fruit varying from yellow to orangey red. Mandarin is the same species as tangerine; they are remarkably similar and can be interchanged.

BLENDING PROFILE

Mandarin blends well with other citrus oils and spice oils, also neroli, lavender, sandalwood, petitgrain, melissa, ylang ylang, juniper berry, geranium, rosewood, and cypress.

TRADITIONAL USES

Native to China and Southeast Asia, mandarin was sometimes used alongside sweet orange in folk remedies. Today, it is widely used in the flavoring industry, usually in combination with other citrus oils.

THERAPEUTIC PROPERTIES

Antidepressant, anti-inflammatory, antioxidant, antiseptic, antispasmodic, calming, carminative, cholagogue, depurative, digestive, diuretic, sedative, and tonic. *(See glossary on page 158.)*

Safe in pregnancy

Mandarin is safe in pregnancy and is particularly recommended for children to soothe restlessness and agitation. The lovely soft, fruity fragrance is often well

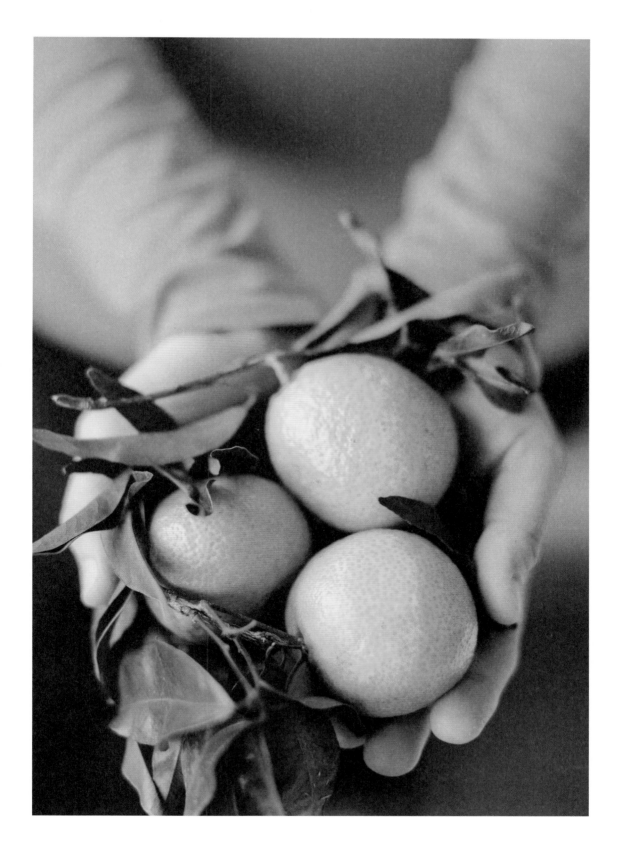

tolerated and enjoyed by women during pregnancy, which is a time when the sense of smell is heightened and many essential oils are not appreciated, or actively cause nausea. One of the best and safest massage blends for pregnant women is to use mandarin blended with neroli.

Blended with lavender and neroli in apricot kernel oil, mandarin helps reduce stretch marks when massaged daily into the abdomen from the fifth month until childbirth. Alternatively, you can make a simple body butter by melting shea butter and adding apricot kernel oil and a few drops of mandarin and neroli; this would make a lovely gift for a pregnant friend.

Gentle tonic

Overall, mandarin is uplifting, cheering, and soothing. This makes it a useful choice in blends to counteract depression and stress, particularly when blended with jasmine, Roman chamomile, or rose. Mandarin has a tonic effect on the digestion system, and is good for all digestive upsets. It is also effective in blends with other citrus oils and detoxifying oils, such as juniper berry and sweet fennel, to help improve circulation of the lymph system.

It makes a pleasant addition to all massage blends and perfumes, bringing a light, gentle, calming note. Psychologically, mandarin is strengthening, and has a slight hypnotic quality, helping switch off an overactive mind, and promoting restful sleep. Mandarin has a soft, delicate quality that helps people connect with their inner child.

Mandarin pomander

In the Middle Ages oranges, mandarins, and tangerines were often used to make pomanders. A typical pomander would consist of an orange or mandarin studded with cloves, which was held close to the nose to repel bad smells. Pomanders were also useful for fighting off colds, respiratory infections, and even plague. This is because both the cloves and the citrus fruit released their antiseptic and antiviral properties, as well as their pleasant fruity, spicy fragrance. A contemporary version of a pomander still smells good and fends off winter chills and fevers. Pomanders also evoke traditional Christmas aromas.

You will need:

- **1 firm mandarin or small orange**
- **10–20 clove buds**

1. Using the sharp end of the clove, push each clove into the fruit, up to the bud. Stud them evenly over the mandarin. You could also add some cinnamon sticks or star anise for a festive fragrance.

2. Place your pomander on a decorative dish and let the aroma perfume your home and fend off germs.

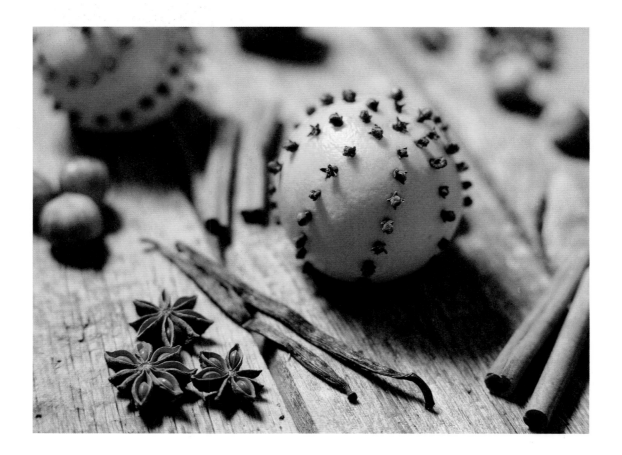

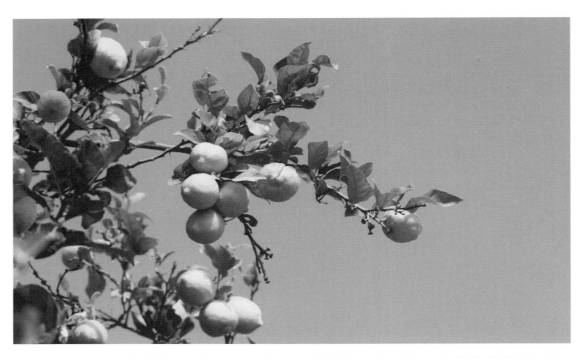

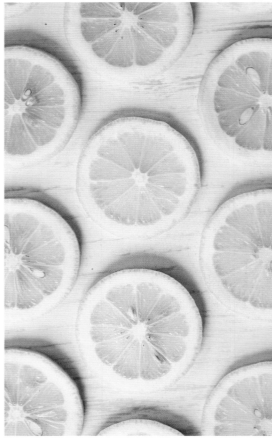

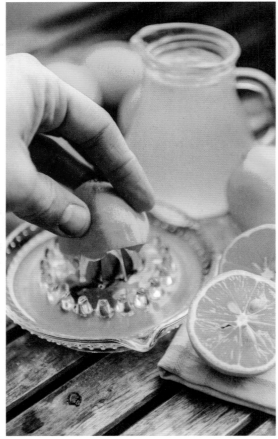

LEMON

Citrus limonum

*Botanical Family:
Rutaceae*

The fresh smell of lemon helps spring clean the mind. Great to use on busy days, lemon brings clarity and mental focus.

METHOD OF EXTRACTION:
Cold pressed. The peel of the nearly ripe and ripe fruit is mechanically squeezed to express the essential oil.

REGIONS OF ORIGIN:
America, China, Cyprus, Israel, Italy, the Middle East, Sicily.

CHARACTERISTICS:
Lemon is a yellow or yellow-green thin essential oil that easily drops from the bottle dropper.

FRAGRANCE DESCRIPTION:
Lemon has clean, fresh, light, sharp top notes with slightly sweet citrussy undertones.

SAFE USAGE: Do not use if you have very sensitive skin, and do not use before exposure to sunlight. Use no more than 3 drops in the bath.

PLANT DESCRIPTION

Lemon is a small evergreen tree, with oval leaves, fragrant flowers, and green fruits that turn yellow as the fruit ripens. The lemon tree typically fruits all year.

BLENDING PROFILE

Lemon blends well with the other citrus and floral oils, and almost all other essential oils. A useful tip: If a blend smells wrong or lacks harmony, add a few drops of lemon, which often improves the overall fragrance.

TRADITIONAL USES

Originally a native of China, the lemon tree came to Europe, via Persia and the Middle East, in the 12th century. Columbus took seeds to the Americas where lemon trees are now cultivated extensively. Traditionally used to combat scurvy in sailors during long sea voyages, lemon juice was also used as a diaphoretic and diuretic. Lemon juice is used to treat hiccups, rheumatism, and even poisoning. Lemon essential oil is used extensively in the flavoring, pharmaceutical, and cosmetics industries.

THERAPEUTIC PROPERTIES

Antiseptic, antimicrobial, antirheumatic, antiseptic, astringent, antispasmodic, bactericide, carminative, cicatrisant, diuretic, depurative, diaphoretic, febrifuge, hemostatic, hypotensive, insecticidal, rubefacient, tonic, and vermifuge. *(See glossary on page 158.)*

Detoxifying and refreshing

Lemon essential oil is useful in many ways. Its hemostatic properties help stop bleeding and, combined with its bactericidal properties, this means lemon is excellent in a wash for cleaning cuts and grazes. It is detoxifying and valuable in lymphatic drainage massage to help combat cellulite. Lemon is a tonic of the circulatory system, it cleanses the blood, and it is also helpful for reducing varicose veins. Its ability to counteract acidity makes lemon useful for alleviating rheumatic conditions, gout, arthritis, and digestive acidity. Overall, lemon is refreshing, purifying, and cleansing.

Skin toning

It is used in skincare to brighten the complexion, and is indicated for oily skin and acne. It also tones aging skin. A drop of neat lemon oil can be applied to heal verrucas and warts. Lemon's antimicrobial properties help the body fight infection, and it is useful in sprays and burners to prevent the spread of infection.

Clarifying and reviving

Psychologically, lemon is radiant, reviving, and stimulating. It lifts the spirits and clears the mind, bringing a calm clarity. Lemon helps prevent emotional outbursts, and assists in making decisions. It sheds light when the mind has become dark, foggy, or confused. Lemon is useful in meditation for clearing the mind, and it also opens the heart.

Lemon curd

Traditionally, lemon curd uses finely grated zest—which contains essential oil—to strengthen the flavor. You can substitute some or all of the zest for lemon essential oil.

You will need:

- 6–8 organic lemons
- 10 drops organic lemon essential oil (optional)
- 1 cup superfine sugar
- 3 eggs
- ½ cup sweet butter, cubed

1. Wash the lemons thoroughly. Cut each fruit in half and squeeze out the juice until you have 6 fl oz (180 ml).

2. Scar the peel with a sharp knife to release the essential oil. Squeeze each lemon peel firmly over a small jug to catch the essential oil; you will not end up with much, but each drop is potent. Use gloves to prevent any lemon essential oil getting on your hands, or wash your hands immediately afterward.

3. Grate 1 teaspoon of zest to add to the lemon curd, if desired. Alternatively, you can use up to 10 drops of organic lemon essential oil.

4. Place all the ingredients in a pan and heat gently. Lightly whisk the mixture for 6–8 minutes until soft peaks begin to form. Remove from the heat and pour into sterilized glass jars. Leave until quite cool then put on lids and store in the fridge.

5. Enjoy on a slice of warm bread!

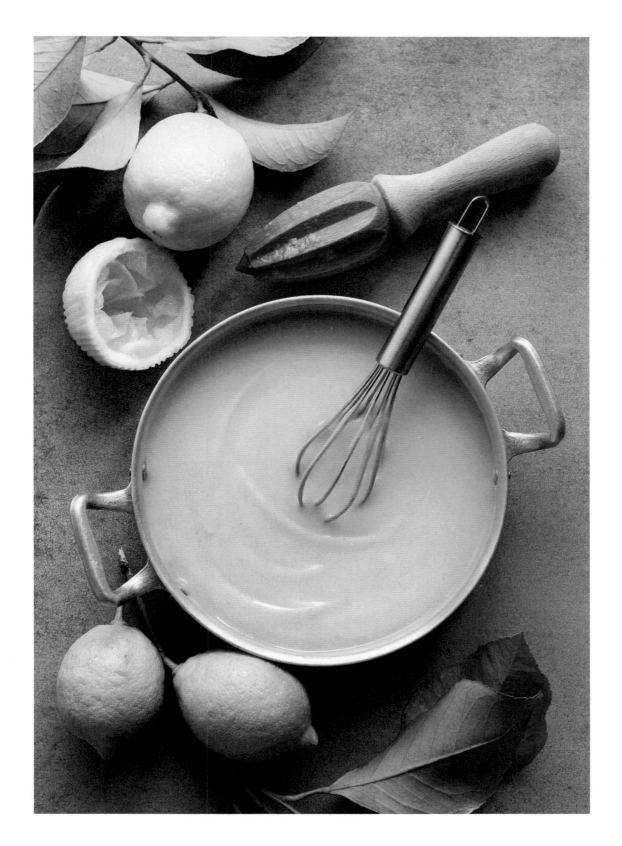

GRAPEFRUIT

Citrus paradisi

Botanical Family:
Rutaceae

Blended with floral and spice oils in massage and bath oils, grapefruit helps to relieve emotional and physical exhaustion. Grapefruit can also improve self-esteem.

METHOD OF EXTRACTION:
Cold pressed. The peel of the nearly ripe grapefruit fruit is mechanically squeezed to express the essential oil.

REGIONS OF ORIGIN:
America, Argentina, Brazil, France, Israel, Nigeria, West Indies.

CHARACTERISTICS:
Grapefruit is a pale orange or clear thin essential oil that easily drops from the bottle dropper.

FRAGRANCE DESCRIPTION:
Grapefruit has clean, fresh, light, tart top notes with sweet citrussy undertones.

SAFE USAGE: Grapefruit is generally a safe essential oil. Use no more than 4–5 drops in the bath.

PLANT DESCRIPTION

Grapefruit is a big tree, growing to about 30 feet. It has glossy green leaves, white flowers, and large fruits. These are either the familiar yellow fruits or the more recently introduced pink grapefruit, which is sweeter and so has become more popular. However, there is little difference in fragrance or properties between the two essential oils.

BLENDING PROFILE

Grapefruit blends well with the other citrus oils and spice oils, and also palmarosa, neroli, rosemary, cypress, geranium, juniper berry, lavender, jasmine, and ylang ylang.

TRADITIONAL USES

Grapefruit is the only citrus fruit native to the New World. It originated in the West Indies before spreading around the globe. There is little indication of traditional use of grapefruit other than as a fruit for eating and juicing. Today, the essential oil is used in the flavor and cosmetic industries. The fruit is also much used in detoxifying diets, as it efficiently cleanses and detoxifies the digestive tract and body.

THERAPEUTIC PROPERTIES

Antidepressant, antiseptic, astringent, antispasmodic, depurative, disinfectant, diuretic, stimulant, and tonic. *(See glossary on page 158.)*

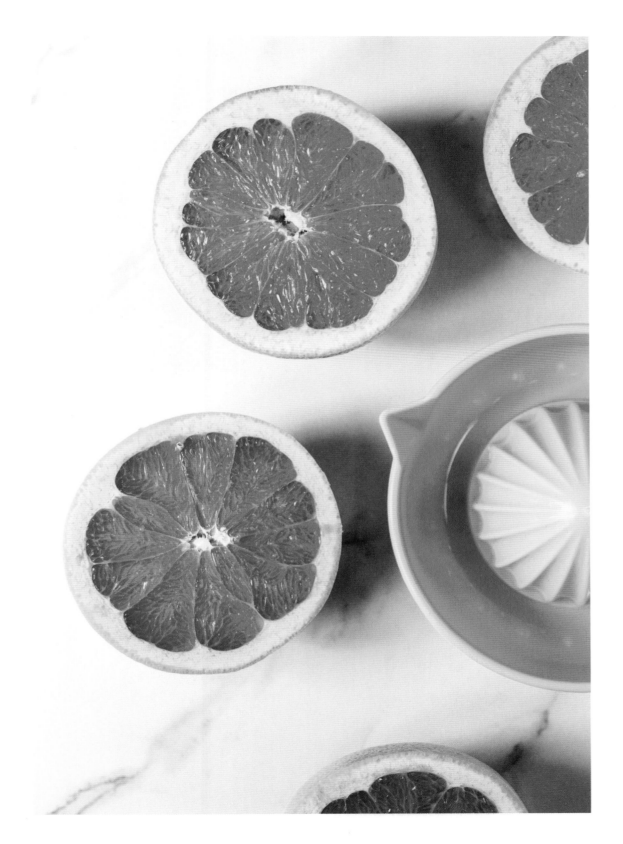

Purifying

Grapefruit has similar properties to the other citrus essential oils. It is useful in lymphatic drainage massage, particularly when blended with rosemary and juniper berry, as it helps alleviate water retention, dispel toxins, and remove cellulite.

Grapefruit is good for a congested or overheated liver and, when added to a morning bath with rosemary, it can help relieve a hangover. It has a tonic effect on the scalp. You can blend it with cedarwood or rosemary and mix into a base shampoo to keep the scalp healthy and dandruff-free. Grapefruit is also useful in skincare, particularly for improving the appearance of oily skin, congested skin, and acne. Overall, grapefruit is uplifting, cleansing, and stimulating.

Promotes optimism

Psychologically, grapefruit is refreshing and reviving, helping alleviate stress, depression, nervous exhaustion, and tension. Grapefruit lifts self-esteem and promotes optimism, creating an overall sunny disposition.

Grapefruit marmalade

This delicious grapefruit marmalade can be made with yellow or pink grapefruit, or a mix of the two varieties.

You will need:

- 2 large or 3 small grapefruit
- 1 extra grapefruit, juiced
- juice of 1 lemon
- 2½ cups light brown sugar
- 2½ cups jam sugar
- 2–3 drops organic grapefruit essential oil (optional)

1. Wash the grapefruit thoroughly and place in a large pan with sufficient water to float. Cover, bring to the boil, and boil for 2 hours. Top up with boiling water, as necessary, to avoid the fruit sticking to the bottom of the pan.

2. Meanwhile, scrub the extra grapefruit, and clean, halve, and extract the juice. Scar the peel with a sharp knife and squeeze out a few drops of essential oil over a small jug. Wear gloves or wash your hands immediately afterward.

3. Remove the fruit from the pan and discard the water. Let the fruit cool and then finely chop.

4. Return the fruit to the pan, along with the lemon juice, sugars, grapefruit juice, and essential oil. Heat gently until the sugars dissolve. Boil for 15 minutes, or until a teaspoon of marmalade dropped onto a cold saucer gels. If you prefer a fine texture, use a blending stick once the sugar has dissolved.

5. Pour into sterilized jars and let cool before putting on the lids. Label and store in the fridge.

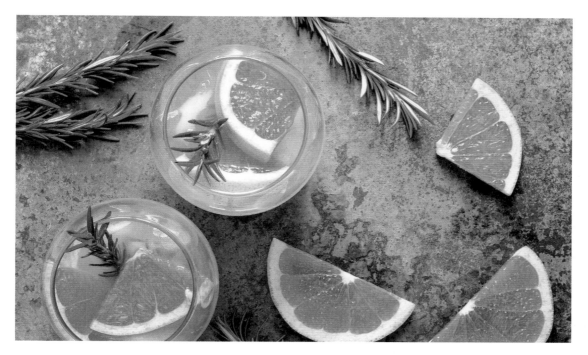

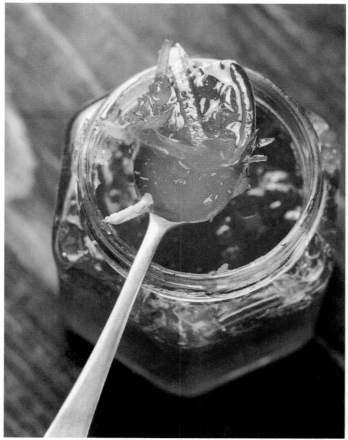

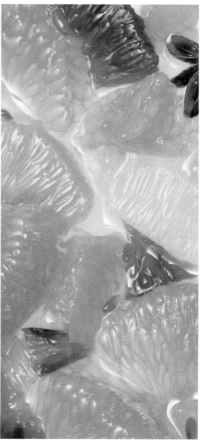

LIME

Citrus aurantifolia

Botanical Family:
Rutaceae

> Psychologically, lime is refreshing and uplifting to the mind and emotions, helping to relieve fatigue, apathy, and depression.

METHOD OF EXTRACTION:
Cold pressed or steam distilled. The peel of the nearly ripe lime fruit is mechanically squeezed to express the essential oil. Occasionally the whole fruit is steam distilled.

REGIONS OF ORIGIN:
America, Brazil, Italy, Mexico, Peru, West Indies.

CHARACTERISTICS:
Cold-pressed lime is either a pale or rich olive-green-golden thin essential oil that easily drops from the bottle dropper. Distilled lime is a pale green or clear thin essential oil that easily drops from the bottle dropper.

FRAGRANCE DESCRIPTION:
Cold-pressed lime has a tart lime aroma with clean, fresh, citrus top notes and slightly bitter undertones. Steam-distilled lime has fresh, clean, sour lime top notes, with almost sweet undertones.

PLANT DESCRIPTION

Lime is an evergreen tree growing up to 15 feet. It has drooping branches, smooth oval leaves, small white flowers, and small green fruit. There are many varieties of lime. Originally from Asia, lime is now cultivated in many warm, temperate countries.

BLENDING PROFILE

Lime blends with other citrus oils and spice oils, and also neroli, petitgrain, lavender, geranium, clary sage, ylang ylang, rosemary, cypress, and jasmine.

TRADITIONAL USES

There are two main types of lime: Key West, Indian, and Mexican cultivars; and a Persian cultivar, which is the type usually sold as fresh fruit. Lime originated in north India and spread to Central and South America through trade with the Polynesians. The Arabs took limes, along with other citrus fruits, to the Middle East and to Europe around the 16th century. Ships transporting lime and other citrus fruits were called "lime juicers," as crews relied on limes and lemons to prevent scurvy, as all citrus fruits have high levels of vitamin C.

In contemporary use distilled lime is used to flavor food and beverages, such as ginger ale and cola drinks, and is used in the perfume industry. Cold-pressed lime is used in men's toiletries and perfumery.

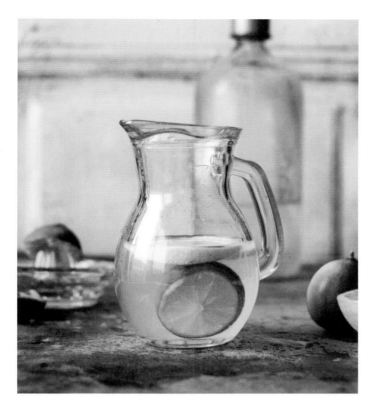

THERAPEUTIC PROPERTIES

Antiseptic, antiviral, astringent, aperitif, bactericide, disinfectant, febrifuge, hemostatic, insecticide, restorative, and tonic. *(See glossary on page 158.)*

Revitalizing

Lime revitalizes a tired mind, alleviates anxiety and adds an interesting fresh, clean, sharp note to perfumes and massage blends. Lime has a similar action to other citrus oils, especially lemon. It is useful in lymphatic-drainage massage to alleviate cellulite and fluid retention and improve poor circulation. It can also help with weight loss and skin toning. Lime has an astringent action, which helps treat oily skin, clogged pores, and acne by counteracting overproduction of sebum.

Immuno-stimulant

Useful to cool fevers, lime's antimicrobial properties also help stimulate the immune system. Lime helps ease coughs, bronchitis, sore throats, and sinusitis. Lime can help alleviate the symptoms of arthritis and rheumatism, relieving pain in muscles and joints, as it helps clear out toxins and congestion. For these conditions local massage is best, with blends including lime, although it's important to gently exercise the joints afterwards. Lime has a tonic restorative action and is good to use in convalescence, especially after a long illness or for chronic debility.

SWEET MARJORAM

Origanum majorana

Botanical Family:
Lamiaceae (Labiatae)

Sweet marjoram is the great comforter of essential oils. The plant is renowned for its versatility because all forms of the herb are warming, fortifying, and soothing.

METHOD OF EXTRACTION:
The essential oil is steam distilled from the dried leaves and flowering tops.

REGIONS OF ORIGIN:
Bulgaria, Egypt, France, Germany, Hungary, Italy, Morocco, Poland, Tunisia, Turkey.

CHARACTERISTICS:
Sweet marjoram is a pale yellow to amber thin oil that easily drops from the bottle dropper.

FRAGRANCE DESCRIPTION:
Sweet marjoram has spicy, herbaceous top notes with warm, woody, camphoraceous undertones.

SAFE USAGE: Avoid during the first three months of pregnancy.

PLANT DESCRIPTION

Sweet marjoram is a tender, bushy perennial herb growing up to 2 feet. It is usually cultivated as an annual in colder climates. A strongly fragrant bush, sweet marjoram has dark green leaves, a hairy stem, and clusters of white flowers.

BLENDING PROFILE

Sweet marjoram blends well with other herbal oils, also lavender, bergamot, cypress, chamomile, juniper berry, geranium, and eucalyptus.

TRADITIONAL USES

Sweet marjoram is native to the Mediterranean region and has been used since ancient times in medicine and cooking. The Greeks called sweet marjoram the funeral herb and planted it on graves to bring spiritual peace to the dead. In Europe, Culpepper recommended sweet marjoram for chest, liver, and menstrual ailments. It was also used for respiratory and digestive complaints, as well as for muscle and joint aches and pains.

In medieval Europe, sweet marjoram was often used as a strewing herb to cover and warm floors in winter and offer defense against bad smells, germs, and insects. Today, sweet marjoram is used in the pharmaceutical and flavoring industries.

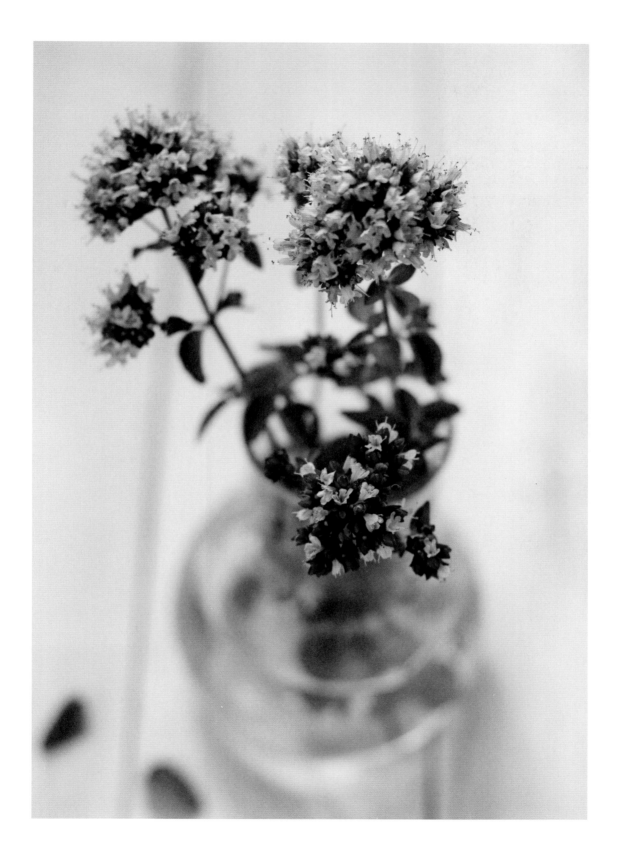

THERAPEUTIC PROPERTIES

Analgesic, antiseptic, antispasmodic, anaphrodisiac, antiviral, bactericide, carminative, cordial, digestive, diuretic, emmenagogue, expectorant, hypotensor, nervine, sedative, stomachic, tonic, vasodilator, and vulnerary. *(See glossary on page 158.)*

Warming and comforting
Sweet marjoram warms and comforts mind, emotions, spirit, and body, and is especially good for grief, soothing, and giving solace to the heart and emotions. However, the effects of sweet marjoram can be numbing, and it must be used with caution. This quality is reflected in its anaphrodisiac quality, which means the lessening, or numbing, of sexual desire. However, for those who choose celibacy, for religious or other reasons, this can be a useful property. Overall, sweet marjoram is fortifying, warming, and comforting.

Relieves pain
Useful for relaxing tight, stiff muscles, and easing rheumatic pain, sweet marjoram is excellent in massage, gently dilating blood vessels to produce a local warming effect. Sweet marjoram is also good in the bath, but works best blended with lavender or other sweeter essential oils. It also works well in a hot compress over painful joints. Sweet marjoram stimulates and strengthens peristalsis so is good for relieving constipation, flatulence, and colic when used in local abdominal massage, particularly when blended with sweet orange and black pepper.

Used in a hot compress, blended with lavender, chamomile, or clary sage, sweet marjoram relieves menstrual cramps. It is useful in an inhalation or chest rub for respiratory complaints, such as colds, flu, bronchitis, emphysema, and whooping cough. For these conditions, sweet marjoram works best when blended with eucalyptus, ravintsara, tea tree, and lavender.

Sweet marjoram is useful in a hot compress on the back of the neck, along with a cold compress of lavender on the forehead, to relieve headaches. These are often caused by constricted blood flow, usually brought on by stress and tension.

Eases stress
Psychologically, sweet marjoram acts like a second skin, calming oversensitivity, and easing stress and nervous tension. Sweet marjoram offers comfort to the sad and lonely, and it is comforting and reassuring emotionally for those who are celibate. It helps the flow of subtle energy throughout the body, and brings out hidden strength and endurance.

Sweet marjoram massage blend

This comforting, pain-relieving oil can be massaged gently over the abdomen to soothe menstrual cramps, digestive pain, and constipation. It's important to massage in a clockwise direction, as this follows the direction of the digestive system.

The massage oil also helps soothe sore muscles, and rheumatic or arthritic joints.

You will need:

- 2 tsp sweet almond oil
- 2 drops sweet marjoram essential oil
- 2 drops chamomile essential oil
- 1 drop lavender essential oil
- 1 drop black pepper essential oil

1. Measure the sweet almond oil into a small dish and add the correct number of drops for each essential oil. Mix well and massage as required.

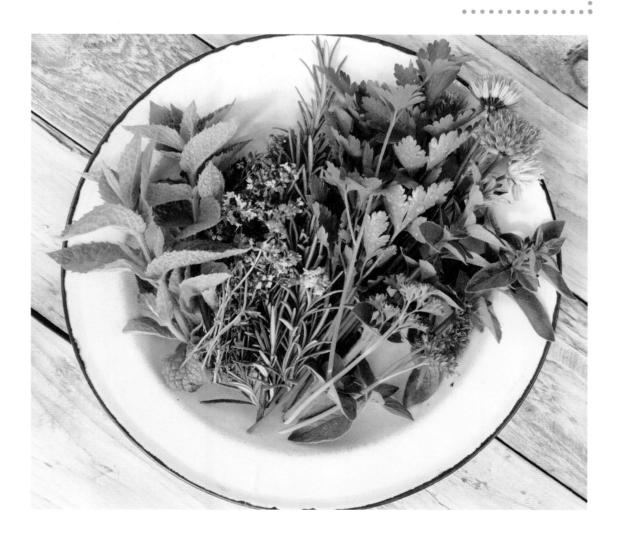

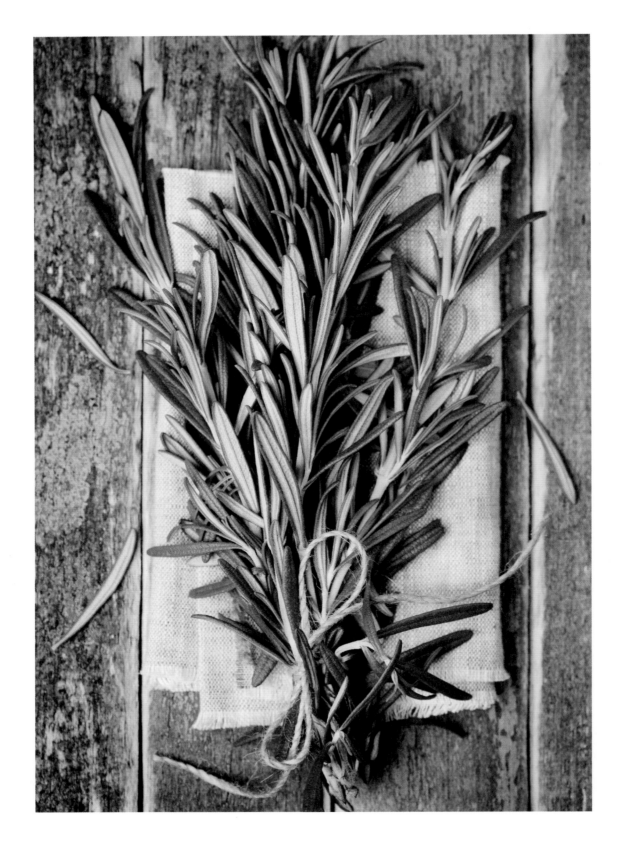

ROSEMARY

Rosmarinus officinalis

Botanical Family:
Lamiaceae (Labiatae)

Rosemary is a popular aromatic herb and has been used widely in food and medicine for thousands of years.

METHOD OF EXTRACTION:
Rosemary essential oil is steam distilled from the fresh flowering tops. Sometimes the twigs and branches are included, but this produces a poorer-quality oil.

REGIONS OF ORIGIN:
California, Corsica, England, France, Portugal, Russia, Spain, Tunisia.

CHARACTERISTICS:
Rosemary is a pale yellow or almost colorless, clear, thin oil that easily drops from the bottle dropper.

FRAGRANCE DESCRIPTION:
Rosemary has fresh, green top notes with herbaceous, balsamic, woody, and camphoraceous undertones.

SAFE USAGE: Avoid during the first three months of pregnancy, and do not use on those who suffer from epilepsy.

PLANT DESCRIPTION

Rosemary is an aromatic, perennial, shrubby bush that grows up to 6 feet with silver-green needle-like leaves, and distinctive, prolific sky-blue flowers.

BLENDING PROFILE

Rosemary blends well with most spice oils, also lavender, bergamot, basil, frankincense, juniper berry, pine needles, thyme, melissa, cedarwood, lemon, citronella, lemongrass, and petitgrain.

TRADITIONAL USES

Native to the Mediterranean, rosemary has been used since ancient times. The name comes from *ros* meaning dew and *marinus* meaning sea, as rosemary typically grows near the coast. The Greeks and Romans considered rosemary a sacred plant symbolizing love and death. Medicinally, Dioscorides suggested it for stomach and liver problems, Hippocrates for liver and spleen disorders, and Galen for jaundice. Rosemary was burned with juniper as cheap incense to purify the air and prevent infection, and it was used in French hospitals until the end of the 19th century. Culpepper recognized it as a mental stimulant and suggested it for giddiness and loss of memory. Rosemary has frequently been used as a hair and scalp tonic to help restore hair loss, tone the scalp, and prevent dandruff. Pre-refrigeration, rosemary was used to help preserve meat.

THERAPEUTIC PROPERTIES

Analgesic, antidepressant, antiseptic, antispasmodic, astringent, carminative, cephalic, cholagogue, digestive, diuretic, emmenagogue, hepatic, hypertensor, nervine, rubefacient, stimulant, sudorific, and tonic. *(See glossary on page 158.)*

Reviving and refreshing

Rosemary is the strongest cephalic, or mental stimulant, essential oil, and scientifically proves correct the old folk saying: "Rosemary for remembrance." A classic remedy is 1 drop of rosemary mixed with 2 drops of neroli dabbed on the wrists before taking an exam; neroli calms the nerves and rosemary strengthens the mind and increases creativity. Overall, rosemary is reviving, refreshing, and strengthening.

Rosemary is good for strengthening the liver and gall bladder. It is a heart tonic that can be used to help cardiac fatigue and heart palpitations. It is also helpful to raise low blood pressure and to stimulate poor circulation of the hands and feet. Rosemary is recommended for its mucolytic properties and is useful in inhalations for bronchitis, sinusitis, and asthma.

An effective antiseptic

Excellent and much used in massage, rosemary helps to relax tight, overworked muscles, relieve fluid retention, and detoxify the lymphatic system. Reputed to help hair growth, it makes a good tonic for the scalp and hair. As an effective antiseptic, rosemary used in a burner can help prevent the spread of airborne infections. It is also a powerful liver tonic: 3 drops of rosemary mixed with 3 drops of grapefruit in a morning bath can help relieve a hangover swiftly. It helps to deter insects, especially when mixed with citronella.

Aids meditation

Psychologically, rosemary is stimulating, purifying, and protecting. It is a common ingredient in incense and aids meditation, keeping the mind clear and alert. Eau de Cologne is traditionally made from essential oils of bergamot, neroli, lavender, and rosemary. Other citrus oils and petitgrain may be included, and occasionally thyme replaces rosemary. It is a psychic protector, a symbol of friendship and love, and was traditionally burned at weddings and funerals. Rosemary is associated with the third-eye chakra, assisting clear thought and inner vision.

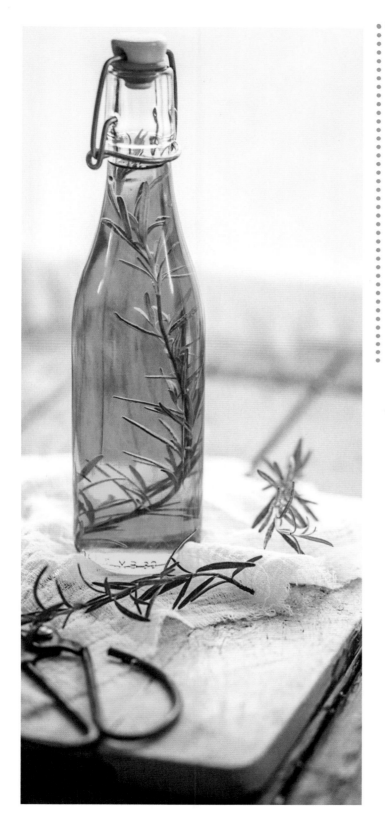

Rosemary-infused olive oil

Use this fragrant and delicious oil for roasting vegetables, in salad dressings, and whenever you need a herby oil.

You will need:

- 1 bottle good-quality olive oil, preferably organic
- 1 large sprig of fresh rosemary, washed and dried

1. Pour out a little of the oil and reserve for later use. Then gently insert the sprig of rosemary into the bottle; it might be a bit of a squeeze if the bottle opening is narrow.

2. Let the oil sit for a couple of weeks to allow the rosemary to fully infuse the oil, and then use as desired.

CLARY SAGE

Salvia sclarea

Botanical Family:
Lamiaceae or Labiatae

Clary sage is one of the most valuable essential oils for treating menstrual cramps, and to relax mind, emotions, and body. Use in baths or hot compresses on the abdomen.

METHOD OF EXTRACTION:
Clary sage essential oil is steam distilled from the fresh flowering tops and leaves.

REGIONS OF ORIGIN:
Americas, central Europe, England, France, Morocco, Russia.

CHARACTERISTICS:
Clary sage is a clear or pale-olive thin oil that easily drops from the bottle dropper.

FRAGRANCE DESCRIPTION:
Clary sage has sweet, musky, herbaceous top notes with nutty, almost floral, undertones.

SAFE USAGE: Avoid during pregnancy. Do not use for a few hours before or after drinking alcohol.

PLANT DESCRIPTION

Clary sage is a tall biennial or perennial herb with big, hairy, purple-green leaves, and prolific, small, blue-violet, or white flowers.

BLENDING PROFILE

Clary sage blends well with citrus and other herbal oils, also lavender, coriander, cardamom, frankincense, rose, jasmine, pine needles, geranium, sandalwood, cedarwood atlas, and palmarosa.

TRADITIONAL USES

The English word clary is derived from the Latin *sclarea* meaning clear. This became modified to *clear eye* because infusions of the herb were used to bathe and clean the eyes. Note that this is an infusion of the herb; you would never use essential oils on or near the eyes as they are much too concentrated. Culpepper mentions that compresses of clary sage might reduce tumors and swellings. It was also used to cool inflammation and soothe sore throats. Sometimes used as a substitute for hops in brewing beer, clary sage was also used to adulterate cheap German wine to make it taste like muscatel, hence it was sometimes called muscatel sage. Beer or wine made with clary sage caused people to become drunk more easily, but also gave bad hangovers! It is still recommended not to combine alcohol and clary sage.

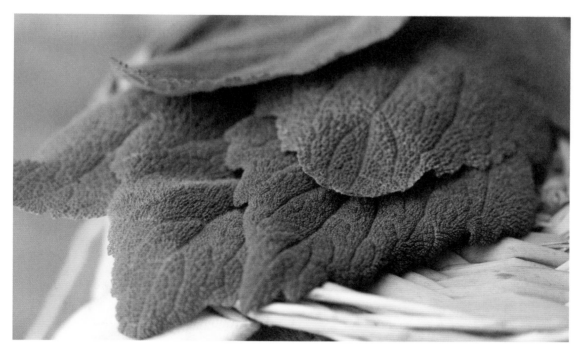

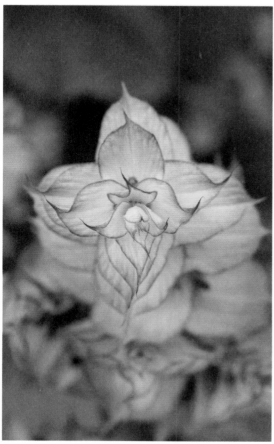

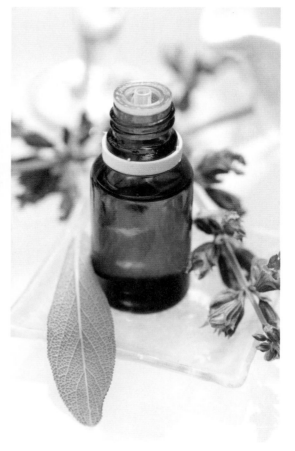

MAIN THERAPEUTIC PROPERTIES

Anticonvulsive, antidepressant, antiseptic, antispasmodic, aphrodisiac, astringent, carminative, deodorant, digestive, emmenagogue, hypotensor, nervine, sedative, and tonic. *(See glossary on page 158.)*

Euphoric and balancing

Clary sage is the most euphoric of the essential oils: In some sensitive people it can produce an almost drug-like narcotic "high." Combined with clary sage's pronounced antidepressant qualities, this euphoria is a potent aid to easing depression, melancholia, anxiety, stress, and chronic general dissatisfaction. Clary sage works mainly by balancing; it is strengthening yet relaxing and promotes harmony. Overall, clary sage is intoxicating, sensuous, and uplifting.

Clary sage is good in a local massage oil over the chest and back to help relieve asthma. Added to hair products or massaged into the scalp it helps prevent dandruff and as it balances sebum levels, it is beneficial for all skin and hair types. Used in a foot bath or bath, and blended with cypress, clary sage helps reduce excessive sweating.

Regulates menstruation

Clary sage eases pain and the estrogenic action from its phytohormones helps bring on and regulate menstruation. Phytohormones are ingredients in plants, mainly herbs, that mimic the action of human hormones. This quality also means clary sage can help treat menopausal symptoms, and can aid childbirth used in a massage oil over the lower back during early labor. Clary sage is a quite powerful aphrodisiac, and is especially good for those who are so stressed out that their sexuality has diminished.

Vivid dreams

Psychologically, clary sage is deeply relaxing, euphoric, and revitalizing. Used in small quantities, it is a useful aid to meditation, and facilitates dream work by encouraging powerful and vivid dreams. Clary sage helps strengthen subtle energies and encourage divine inspiration.

Clary sage hair tonic

Added to conditioner, clary sage helps combat greasy hair. It also stimulates the scalp and reinvigorates hair growth. Clary sage also helps prevent dandruff. Available from health stores, base conditioner is made from natural ingredients with no added color or perfume, and used as a base for your own blends.

You will need:

- 7 fl oz (200 ml) bottle of base conditioner
- 15 drops clary sage essential oil
- 10 drops cedarwood atlas essential oil
- 5 drops sandalwood essential oil
- 3 drops bergamot essential oil
- 2 drops lavender essential oil
- 5 drops rosemary essential oil

1. Pour the conditioner into a jug and add the correct amount of drops of the essential oils. Mix in thoroughly but gently with a chopstick, glass stirring rod or similar to prevent creating air bubbles.

2. Pour back in the bottle and label with the ingredients, amounts, and date.

3. Use the conditioner as desired, working thoroughly into the scalp and hair; leave for up to 5 minutes before rinsing out.

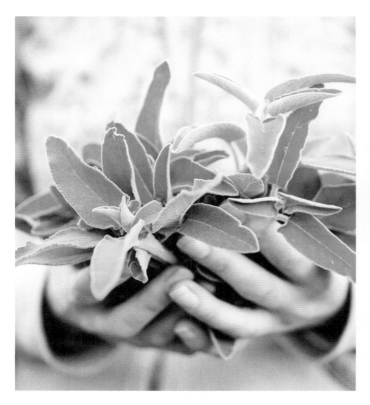

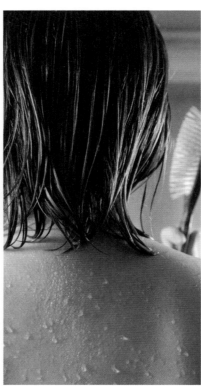

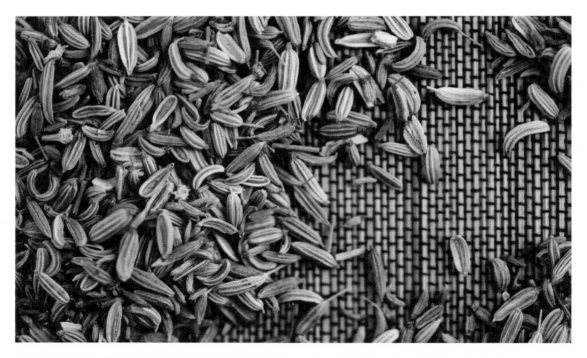

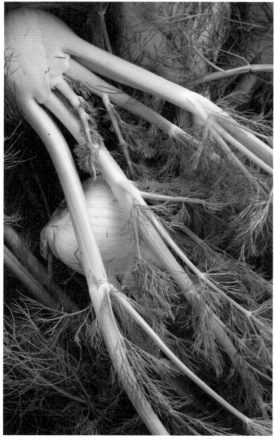

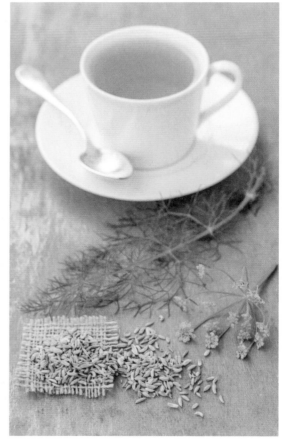

SWEET FENNEL

Foeniculum vulgare

Botanical Family:
Apiaceae (Umbelliferae)

Sweet fennel is one of the best detoxifying essential oils, and is a good choice to use in lymphatic drainage massage.

METHOD OF EXTRACTION:
Sweet fennel essential oil is steam distilled from the crushed seeds.

REGIONS OF ORIGIN:
France, Greece, Italy.

CHARACTERISTICS:
Sweet fennel is a clear to pale yellow thin to viscous oil that easily drops from the bottle dropper.

FRAGRANCE DESCRIPTION:
Sweet fennel has clean, sweet, aniseed top notes with earthy, spicy, peppery undertones.

SAFE USAGE: Avoid during pregnancy, and do not use on those with epilepsy.

PLANT DESCRIPTION

Sweet fennel is a biennial or perennial herb growing up to 6 feet, with distinctive, delicate feathery leaves, and golden flowers. It's important to distinguish sweet fennel from common or bitter fennel, which usually grows wild, and Florence fennel, which is a smaller plant with a large edible root.

BLENDING PROFILE

Sweet fennel blends well with geranium, lavender, black pepper, rosemary, sandalwood, clary sage, lemon, and cardamom.

TRADITIONAL USES

Native to the Mediterranean region the ancient Egyptians, Greeks, and Romans cultivated sweet fennel for its fruits and edible shoots. The Greeks recognized it as an aid to slimming and believed it conferred longevity, strength, and courage. Marching soldiers and people fasting chewed the seeds to relieve hunger.

Sweet fennel was associated with witchcraft in the Middle Ages in Europe and it was used alongside St John's Wort to protect against evil spirits. Bunches of sweet fennel were commonly hung over doorways to prevent evil spirits from entering. Cole and Culpepper both wrote of the properties of sweet fennel as a digestive. It is used in Traditional Chinese Medicine to treat snakebite. Both Eastern and Western herbalists consider sweet fennel good for liver, spleen, gall bladder, and all manner of digestive complaints. It is an ingredient of children's gripe water and soothes colic. The seeds are widely used as a culinary aid, and the oil is used to flavor toothpastes, bakery items, confectionery, and liqueurs.

THERAPEUTIC PROPERTIES

Antiseptic, antispasmodic, carminative, depurative, diuretic, emmenagogue, expectorant, galactagogue, splenic, and stomachic. *(See glossary on page 158.)*

Purifying and diuretic
Sweet fennel particularly helps alleviate fluid retention, and the often accompanying cellulite and possibly obesity. Its diuretic qualities help rid the body of toxins generally, and it is a good urinary tract antiseptic, in particular, so helpful to treat urinary tract infections and cystitis. Sweet fennel is also excellent for alleviating flatulence and digestive problems. For all digestive issues, local massage with sweet fennel essential oil in the blend, combined with drinking fennel herbal tea, is recommended. Overall, sweet fennel is cleansing, purifying, and revitalizing.

Beneficial during menopause
As a galactagogue, sweet fennel helps produce breast milk, and the presence of phyothormones means it can help regulate the menstrual cycle and reduce the fluctuation of hormones during menopause. Sweet fennel is recommended to relieve catarrh and congestion of the upper respiratory tract. It can help in the treatment of dull and oily skin helping refresh and revitalize the complexion, but needs to be blended carefully owing to its potent aroma.

Psychologically, sweet fennel is protecting, warming, and grounding. A couple of drops of sweet fennel rubbed between the palms and brushed over the aura can protect against psychic disturbance.

Detoxifying massage blend

Sweet fennel can help reduce cellulite and stimulate weight loss; it is most effective when used together with dietary and lifestyle modifications and exercise.

You will need:

- 1 x 1 fl oz (20 ml) dark glass bottle
- 1 fl oz (20 ml) sweet almond oil
- 3 drops sweet fennel essential oil
- 3 drops juniper berry essential oil
- 2 drops grapefruit essential oil
- 2 drops rosemary essential oil

1. Mix the essential oils thoroughly into the almond oil and pour into the bottle. Label the bottle with ingredients, amounts used, and the date.

2. For at least a week, adapt your diet to eliminate salt, sugar, refined food, alcohol, and caffeine; replace with whole grains, fresh fruit and vegetables, fennel tea, and water. Exercise briskly for at least 20 minutes daily. Before bathing or showering, use a soft bath brush in circular movements over the dry skin on your hips, buttocks, stomach, and thighs. Once a day massage a little oil briskly over the same body areas. During the week you may have headaches, which are a side effect of the detoxifying process. After a week you should notice your cellulite has reduced, you have lost weight, and your skin and eyes are clear and bright.

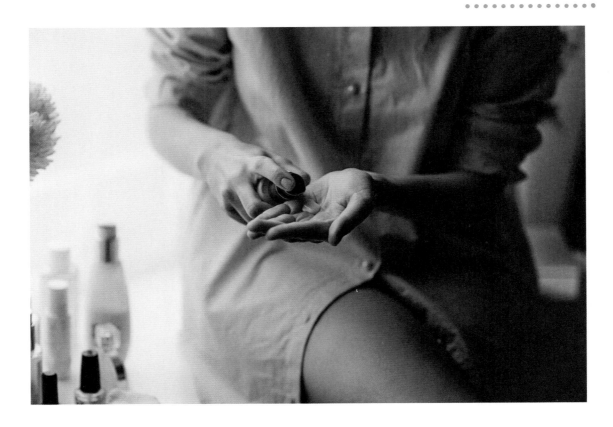

PEPPERMINT

Mentha piperita L.

Botanical Family:
Lamiaceae (Labiatae)

Peppermint has always been used in many different cultures as a remedy for digestive upsets and in dental preparations.

METHOD OF EXTRACTION:
The essential oil is steam distilled from partially dried flowering tops and leaves.

REGIONS OF ORIGIN:
Americas, Australia, Brazil, Bulgaria, China, England, France, Germany, Holland, India, Italy, Morocco, Spain, Tasmania.

CHARACTERISTICS:
Peppermint is a clear to pale yellow thin oil that easily drops from the bottle dropper.

FRAGRANCE DESCRIPTION:
Peppermint has fresh, bright, minty top notes and sharp, grassy, camphoraceous undertones. Spearmint smells softer and sweeter.

SAFE USAGE: Only use 2–3 drops in the bath or in massage oil. Avoid using alongside homeopathic remedies.

PLANT DESCRIPTION

Frequently found in herb gardens, peppermint is a traditional herb in many cultures. Peppermint is a perennial herb with green stems and leaves, and small white flowers. All mints have an invasive root system and are best buried in a strong pot in the ground, or planted in a large garden container.

Other types of mint include spearmint and cornmint, and some of these are also used in aromatherapy. The modern varieties of mint such as pineapple mint, apple mint, and ginger mint are generally not distilled to make essential oil.

BLENDING PROFILE

Peppermint blends well with lavender, rosemary, eucalyptus, and lemon, but its powerful aroma can be difficult to blend successfully. The softer scent of spearmint blends more easily and works well with other herbal oils.

TRADITIONAL USES

Ancient Greeks and Romans used peppermint in wreaths and headbands at feasts and also for culinary purposes for its flavor. Culpepper refers to peppermint for its excellent digestive properties. The herb was used extensively throughout history in many cultures for medicine and flavoring, but peppermint oil began to

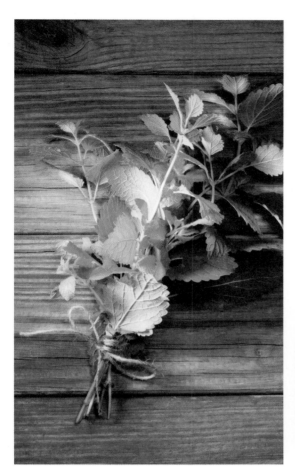
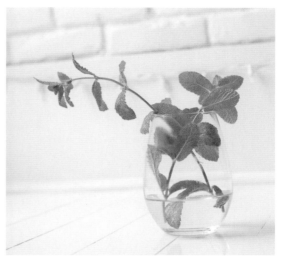
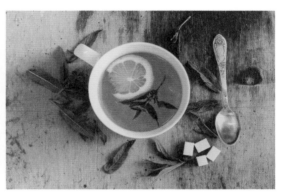
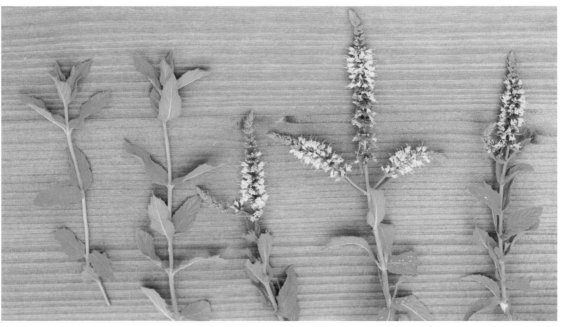

be used only when distillation became widespread. For example, peppermint essential oil arrived in England in the 16th century. Peppermint oil is used extensively in toothpastes and mouthwashes and other toiletries. The herb is widely used as herbal tea.

THERAPEUTIC PROPERTIES

Analgesic, anesthetic, antiseptic, antiphlogistic, antispasmodic, astringent, carminative, cholagogue, cephalic, cordial, decongestant, digestive, expectorant, febrifuge, hepatic, nervine, stimulant, stomachic, sudorific, vasoconstrictor, and vermifuge. *(See glossary on page 158.)*

Stimulating and restorative

Peppermint is one of the best essential oils for all types of digestive upsets, but should be used in a low-percentage dilution—1% or maximum 2% in massage oil—gently massaged over the abdomen in a clockwise direction. Drinking peppermint tea at the same time creates a harmonious synergy between the two forms of peppermint. Overall, peppermint is refreshing, stimulating, and restorative.

Combined with lavender, peppermint helps prevent colds and flu, but use no more than 3 drops in the bath, or in a massage oil or steam inhalation, as it is so strong. Peppermint helps clear the sinuses and may counteract infection. It's good in a facial steam to deeply cleanse and decongest the skin, especially if acne is present. Combined with lavender in cold compresses, peppermint relieves headaches and migraines. It is also a useful general analgesic for myalgia and neuralgia.

Dispels mental fatigue

Peppermint tea can be used as tonic of the spleen and cleanser of the lymphatic system. Vaporized in an essential oil diffuser, peppermint is a powerful cephalic and helps clear a stuffy head and dispel mental fatigue, promoting clear thinking. It stimulates circulation and calms the nerves.

Psychologically, peppermint is bold, promoting clarity and alertness. A few drops sniffed from a tissue may alleviate the symptoms of shock. Peppermint helps lessen feelings of inferiority and insecurity, and can deepen intuitive insight.

Peppermint foot scrub

Peppermint essential oil is excellent in foot scrubs and foot lotions because it is astringent, stimulating, and refreshing to this often-neglected area of the body, and is particularly good for tired feet.

You will need:

- 9 oz (250 g) foaming bath butter
- 1 tbsp almond oil
- 6–8 drops peppermint essential oil
- 1–2 tsp apricot kernel powder (or other exfoliants, such as ground pumice, jojoba beads, or bamboo powder)

1. Blend the foaming bath butter for 2 minutes with an electric hand mixer until increased in size and fluffy.

2. Gradually add the almond oil. Make sure you scrape the sides of the bowl so you mix the butter and oil fully.

3. Add the peppermint oil and the apricot kernel powder, and mix until fully combined. Spoon into jars or other lidded containers.

4. Use your hands or an exfoliating mitt to work the scrub into your feet—it will foam like soap—and then rinse off. Your feet will be deeply cleansed and exfoliated and feel beautifully smooth.

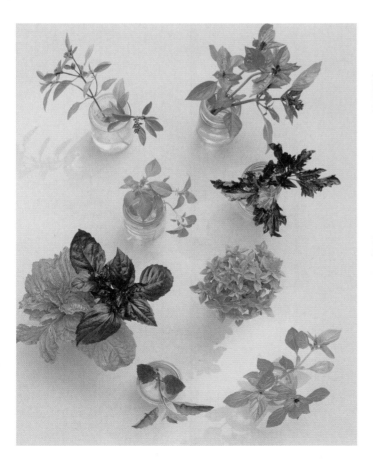

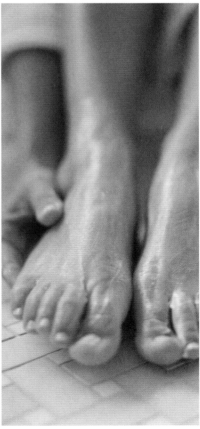

SANDALWOOD

Santalum album, Santalum spicatum, Santalum austrocaledonian

Botanical Family:
Santalaceae

Sandalwood's warm, heavy fragrance increases over time, and it has the longest-lasting aroma of all essential oils. Excellent for nervous tension and depression, it is also a powerful aphrodisiac.

METHOD OF EXTRACTION:
Sandalwood essential oil is steam or water distilled from the powdered heartwood and major roots.

REGIONS OF ORIGIN:
Mysore (India), western and southern Australia.

CHARACTERISTICS:
Sandalwood is a pale yellow viscous oil that easily drops from the dropper insert.

FRAGRANCE DESCRIPTION:
Indian sandalwood has sweet, woody, rose-like top notes and deep, soft, balsamic, spicy, oriental undertones. Australian sandalwood has pronounced resinous, spicy top notes and sweet, dry woody, balsamic undertones.

SAFE USAGE: Sandalwood is a safe essential oil.

PLANT DESCRIPTION

Sandalwood is an evergreen tree with pinky purple flowers reaching up to 38 feet on full maturity at around 60 years old. Mysore in India used to be the main source of sandalwood essential oil. However, owing to the overproduction of Indian sandalwood, *santalum album* became endangered. Indian sandalwood is generally regarded as the finest of the sandalwood oils, but Australian sandalwood varieties—*santalum spicatum* and *santalum austrocaledonian*—are also widely used these days. They have a less fine fragrance, but their therapeutic properties are similar to those of Indian sandalwood.

BLENDING PROFILE

Sandalwood blends well with most floral, herbal and resin oils, also ginger, black pepper, cypress, vetivert, patchouli, petitgrain, and bergamot.

TRADITIONAL USES

Sandalwood timber has always been popular for making furniture, religious, and secular ornaments, and in top-grade incense. The essential oil has long been valued in Ayurvedic medicine. Native Australian aboriginals used to prepare a cough remedy by soaking the bark of Australian sandalwood in boiling water. The seeds were used to alleviate colds and stiffness. Sandalwood oil is extensively used in the cosmetic, pharmaceutical, and

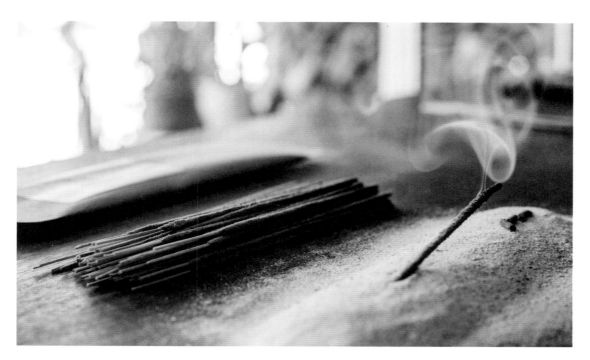

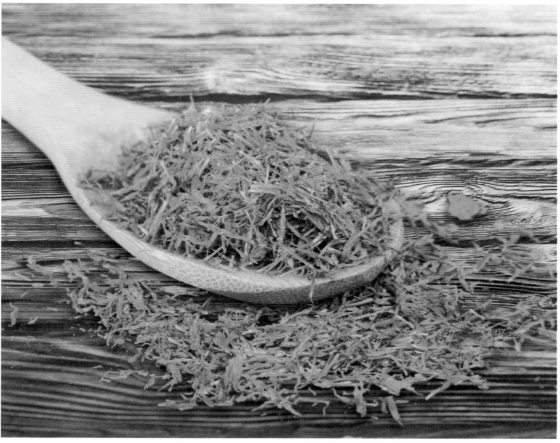

perfumery industries, as the gentle erotic fragrance appeals to women and men, and it is the most tenacious of all essential oils.

THERAPEUTIC PROPERTIES

Antidepressant, anti-inflammatory, antiseptic, antispasmodic, aphrodisiac, astringent, bactericide, carminative, cicatrisant, demulcent, diuretic, expectorant, sedative, and tonic. *(See glossary on page 158.)*

Soothes respiratory complaints

Sandalwood is first choice for chronic bronchitis, soothing and alleviating the symptoms, and is useful for all respiratory complaints, including asthma: It can be used in inhalations, and both local and full body massage. Sandalwood is wonderful in skincare for all skin types, balancing, soothing, and hydrating the skin. It has a rejuvenating effect on mature complexions, and helps treat eczema and psoriasis. It is effective against urinary tract infections. Overall, sandalwood is erotic, relaxing, and uplifting.

Powerful aphrodisiac

Sandalwood is a powerful aphrodisiac, especially useful when sexual problems are caused by stress, anxiety, and isolation. Full-body massage is the best way to utilize the properties of sandalwood. The anti-stress effects of massage, combined with sandalwood, reduce tension and nervousness and work together with sandalwood's aphrodisiac properties to increase desire. Used in massage and baths, sandalwood is cooling and calming, helping prevent tension headaches and effectively relieving insomnia.

Quietens and stills the mind

Psychologically, sandalwood facilitates spiritual practice, and Indian sandalwood has been used in incense as a meditation aid for centuries. It calms irritation born of frustration, quietens and stills the mind, and opens up spiritual potential. Sandalwood is associated with both the crown and base chakras. It is used to arouse kundalini in tantric rituals, meaning it arouses sexual energy for transmutation into spiritual wisdom. Sandalwood helps balance and harmonize the chakras, restoring equilibrium.

Anti-aging face serum

This luxurious serum uses the wonderful rejuvenating effects of sandalwood in combination with other essential and carrier oils, all of which have excellent skincare properties.

You will need:

- 1 x 1 fl oz (20 ml) dark glass bottle
- 1 tsp jojoba oil
- 1 tsp unrefined avocado oil
- 1 tsp cranberry seed oil
- 1 tsp rosehip seed oil
- 2 drops sandalwood essential oil
- 1 drop frankincense essential oil
- 1 drop rose essential oil
- 1 drop patchouli essential oil

1. Measure the jojoba, unrefined avocado, cranberry seed, and rosehip seed oils, and pour into the bottle.

2. Carefully drip in the correct amount of drops of each of the essential oils. Don't be tempted to add more than indicated: at just over 1% dilution this is a safe and effective blend for skin rejuvenation.

3. Gently invert the bottle a few times to mix all the oils thoroughly.

4. Use at night to allow the oils to fully penetrate all layers of the skin, and work their magic while you sleep.

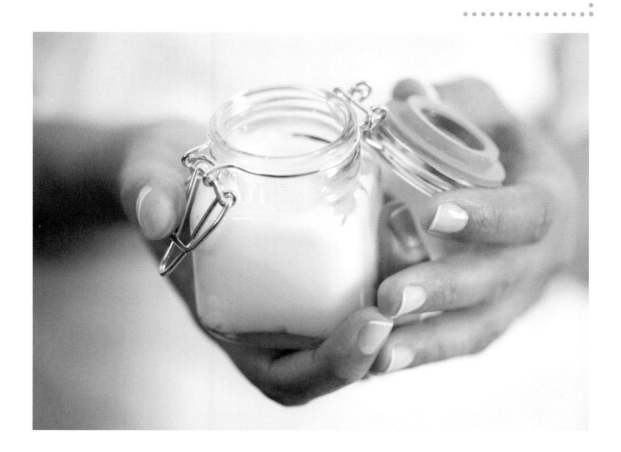

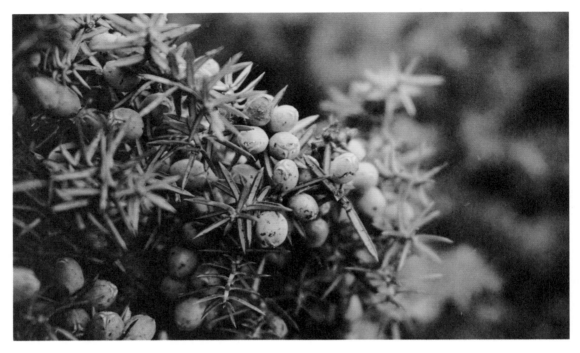

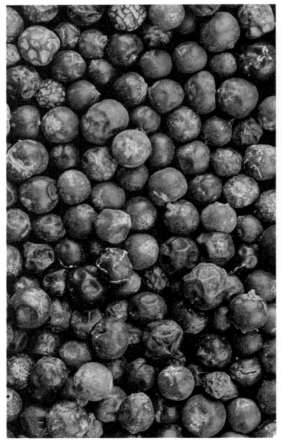

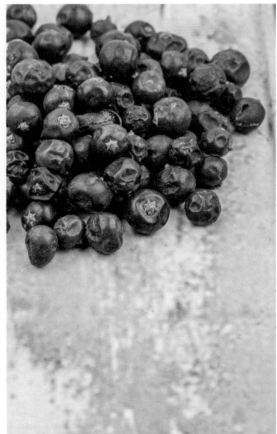

JUNIPER BERRY

Juniperus communis

Botanical Family:
Cupressaceae

The ancient Greeks burned juniper to combat epidemics, while the Tibetans and Native Americans used to burn juniper in traditional ceremonies.

METHOD OF EXTRACTION:
Juniper berry essential oil is steam distilled from the crushed and partly dried ripe berries.

REGIONS OF ORIGIN:
Austria, Canada, Croatia, Czech Republic, France, Hungary, Italy, Serbia.

CHARACTERISTICS:
Juniper berry is a clear or pale green thin oil that easily drops from the bottle dropper.

FRAGRANCE DESCRIPTION:
Jumiper berry has clean, fresh, resinous, turpentine top notes and smoky, balsamic, woody, peppery undertones.

SAFE USAGE: Avoid during pregnancy, and do not use if you have kidney disease. Use in small amounts carefully.

PLANT DESCRIPTION

Juniper is an evergreen tree reaching up to 20 feet high on maturity with blue-green needles, and greeny yellow flowers and berries.

BLENDING PROFILE

Juniper berry blends well with most wood and citrus oils, and also with frankincense, clary sage, rosemary, lavender, geranium, rose, and benzoin.

TRADITIONAL USES

Juniper wood was burned, both as a fumigant and in incense, during religious ceremonies, and as offerings to the gods. Juniper smoke was particularly used to drive away evil spirits and malign influences. The name comes from the Latin *juniores*, meaning young berries. Culpepper recommended juniper for various ailments and the berries were used to treat flatulence, worms, colic, and gastrointestinal infections. Extracts of the berries are used in diuretic and laxative remedies, while the essential oil is used as a fragrance in the pharmaceutical and cosmetics industries. The berries are traditionally used to flavor gin, and generally throughout the flavoring industry.

THERAPEUTIC PROPERTIES

Antiseptic, antirheumatic, antispasmodic, antitoxic, aphrodisiac, astringent, carminative, cicatrisant, depurative, detoxfying, diuretic, emmenagogue, nervine, rubefacient, stimulant, sudorific, tonic, and vulnerary. *(See glossary on page 158.)*

Purifying and restorative

Ensure your juniper oil is extracted from the berries, as this provides the best-quality essential oil. An inferior and harsher essential oil is produced from the needles and twigs, and although cheaper, this oil should be avoided. Juniper berry is one of the best purifying and detoxifying essential oils. On a physical level these qualities manifest as a powerful cleansing and tonic action, making juniper berry very effective in lymphatic drainage massage, and it helps the body eliminate toxins. Juniper berry is also excellent when used for psychic and spiritual purifying. Overall, juniper is cleansing, tonic, and restorative.

Relaxing and warming

One of the best essential oils for cystitis and urinary tract infections, juniper berry is good blended with bergamot in a local wash around the opening of the urethra. Juniper berry helps alleviate nervous tension, intellectual fatigue, and anxiety. Used in small amounts, it is good in skincare, especially when toxins, such as acne, affect the skin. As it is warming, detoxifying, and analgesic, juniper berry is good in massage and hot compresses for aching, overworked muscles, and arthritic or rheumatic joints, including gout.

Clears the mind

Psychologically, juniper berry is purifying, clearing, and fortifying. Traditionally, juniper berry was burned to protect from evil spirits and drive out negative energies, and it is still effective today. A couple of drops rubbed between the palms and brushed over the aura is purifying and protecting. Juniper berry is good in meditation, especially when the mind needs a spring clean. Used in a burner or incense, juniper berry dispels and cleanses the psychic presence of other people.

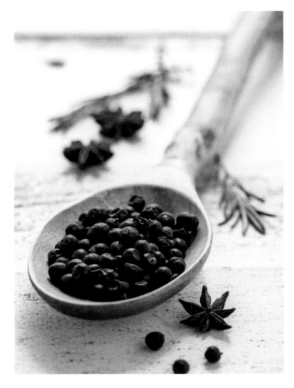

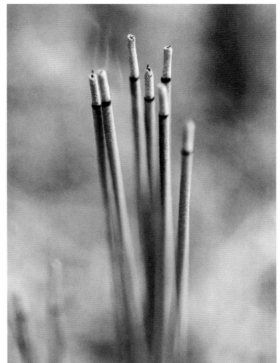

Juniper berry incense

This simple-to-make incense is a lovely way to use juniper berry essential oil in a traditional manner. It is particularly good at psychically cleansing a room.

You will need:

- 1 unscented incense stick (available online or from craft shops)
- 1 x long shallow ceramic or glass dish
- 6 drops juniper berry essential oil
- 6 drops sandalwood essential oil
- 4 drops cypress essential oil
- 2 drops frankincense essential oil
- 2 drops myrrh essential oil

1. Make sure your dish is clean and that the incense stick can lie flat.

2. Place the unscented incense stick in the dish and drop the essential oils along it (don't drop oil on the non-burning, plain end).

3. Gently press the stick and roll it around until it has absorbed all the essential oils. The average stick will absorb up to 20 drops of essential oil.

4. Carefully place the incense stick into a mug or similar container to dry—this will take around 10–15 hours. The stick needs to be completely dry before you burn it.

5. The new incense stick will scent the room you leave it in, so you will have a good idea of what the dry, burning incense will smell like.

CYPRESS

Cupressus sempevirens

Botanical Family:
Cupressaceae

Cypress is good for people who have lost the connection with their sense of harmony and serenity.

METHOD OF EXTRACTION:
The essential oil is steam distilled from the needles and twigs.

REGIONS OF ORIGIN:
Corsica, France, Italy, north Africa, Portugal, Sardinia, Sicily, Spain.

CHARACTERISTICS:
Cypress is a pale yellowish green or colorless thin oil that easily drops from the bottle dropper.

FRAGRANCE DESCRIPTION:
Cypress has spicy, resinous top notes with sweet, smoky, balsamic, woody undertones.

SAFE USAGE: Cypress is a safe essential oil.

PLANT DESCRIPTION

Cypress is an exceptionally long-lived, tall evergreen tree. It grows in a conical shape with graceful slender branches, needles, small flowers, and brown-gray cones or nuts. Cypress trees are often grown near cemeteries. Other varieties of cypress are found around the world, some of which are used to produce essential oil, but the quality of *Cupressus sempevirens* is by far superior to all other varieties.

BLENDING PROFILE

Cypress blends well with most other wood and citrus oils, and also with frankincense, clary sage, lavender, cardamom, sweet marjoram, geranium, neroli, black pepper, and benzoin.

TRADITIONAL USES

Cypress has been used since antiquity by the ancient Egyptians. The ancient Greeks dedicated the cypress tree to Pluto, god of the underworld, hence the practice of planting cypress trees in or nearby to cemeteries. Hippocrates recommended cypress for the treatment of bleeding hemorrhoids. Tibetans use cypress in purification incense, while the Chinese eat the nuts to benefit the liver and respiratory system, and to ameliorate profuse sweating. Cypress is used in the pharmaceutical and perfume industries.

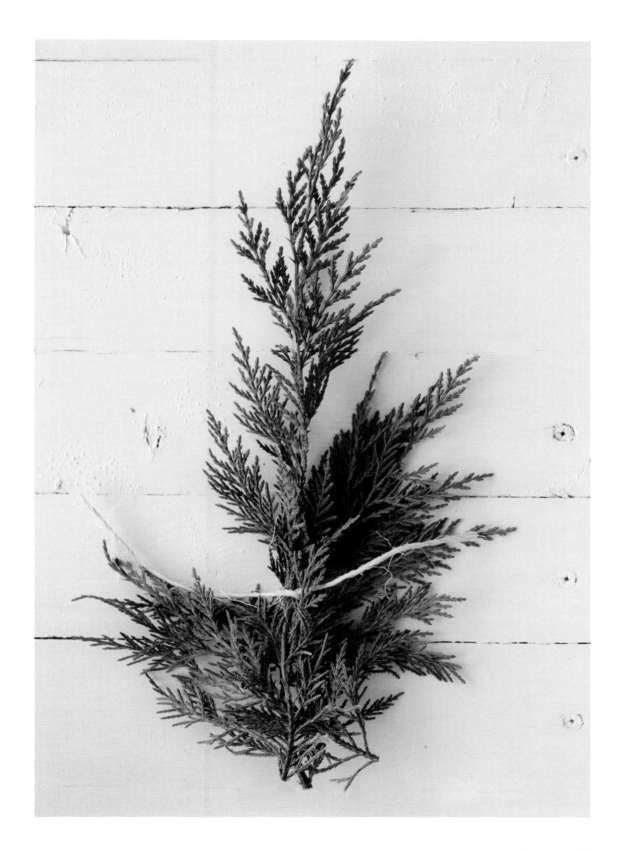

THERAPEUTIC PROPERTIES

Antiseptic, antirheumatic, antispasmodic, antitoxic, antisudorific, astringent, deodorant, diuretic, hepatic, styptic, tonic, and vasoconstrictive. *(See glossary on page 158.)*

A powerful astringent

Cypress is recommended whenever there is excess fluid, as it is a powerful astringent and venous decongestant. This makes cypress first choice (mixed in an ointment) to treat varicose veins and hemorrhoids, and in massage, baths, and compresses to regulate over-heavy and painful menstruation, and reduce edema. Cypress also helps reduce the hot flushes associated with menopause. In a bath or footbath, cypress helps prevent excessive sweating.

The clean, fresh woody aroma of cypress makes it a welcome addition to men's skincare preparations, such as colognes and aftershaves, and it helps ease acne, balance oily and over-hydrated skin. Overall, cypress is warming, drying, and soothing.

Treats coughs and bronchitis

Cypress is effective in inhalations and local massage to treat coughs and bronchitis. It makes a lovely deodorant, blended with bergamot and geranium, dissolved in a little alcohol, and mixed into orange flower water and witch hazel. Cypress helps with nervous weakness and anxiety, restoring a strong, calm demeanor.

Psychic protection

Psychologically, cypress is purifying, protecting, and refreshing, and was traditionally used in different cultures in purifying incense. Like juniper, it provides excellent psychic protection, and as a symbol of eternity, cypress instills strength and wisdom. It improves the flow of stagnant subtle energies. Cypress was dedicated to Pluto, god of the underworld, and so is associated with the base chakra. Cypress can be used in meditations for bereavement, difficult transitions, and painful changes.

Soothing cypress ointment

This simple-to-make healing hemorrhoid ointment is created with a mix of natural oils and waxes, together with cypress and lavender essential oils. It is equally efficacious as a treatment for varicose veins. Ointments are generally greasier than creams, designed for the effective, long-lasting application of active ingredients to the skin surface. They absorb fully into the skin and underlying tissues, but take a longer time to disappear off the surface of the skin.

You will need:

- 2 oz–2¼ oz (50–60 g) dark glass jar
- 2 tbsp olive oil
- 2 tsp calendula infused oil
- 2 g beeswax
- 7 drops cypress essential oil
- 3 drops lavender essential oil

1. Measure the oils and beeswax into a small glass bowl. Place in a shallow pan of simmering water over a low heat. Stir the wax until it is melted and fully integrated with the oils.

2. Remove from the heat and stir gently as the mixture cools. When you notice the mixture is beginning to set, it will turn opaque or milky and gradually start to thicken.

3. Drip in the cypress and lavender oils, stir to mix, and pour into a clean glass jar before the mixture sets.

4. Label the jar with the ingredients and date.

5. Use the cypress ointment as you would a regular hemorrhoid ointment or varicose vein treatment. This homemade cypress ointment is completely natural and safe to use.

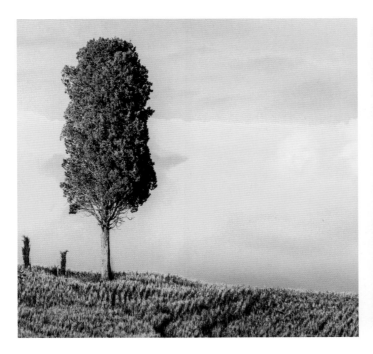

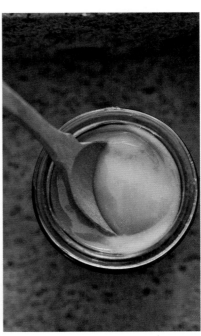

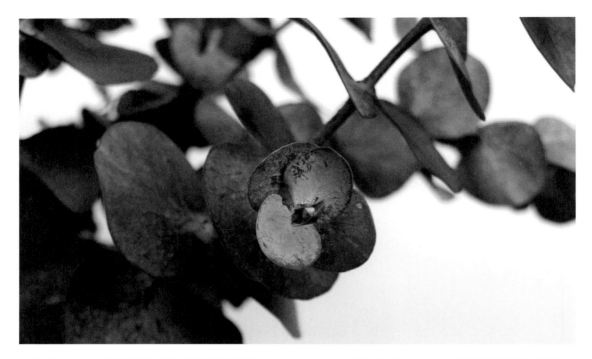

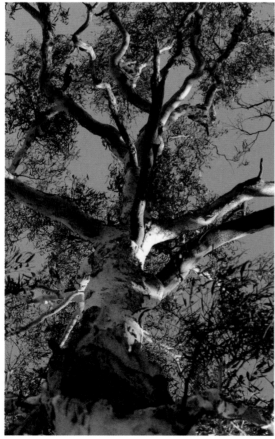

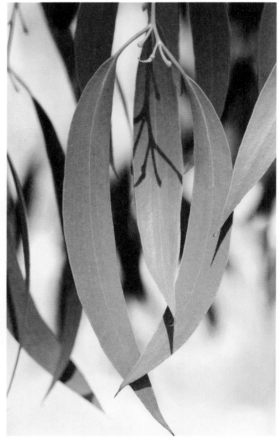

—EUCALYPTUS BLUE GUM—

Eucalyptus globulus

Botanical Family:
Myrtaceae

This stimulating and refreshing antiseptic oil is widely used as a decongestant and is great for clearing the head as well as healing insect bites and stings.

METHOD OF EXTRACTION:
The essential oil is steam distilled from the fresh or partially dried leaves.

REGIONS OF ORIGIN:
Australia, China, Portugal, Spain, Tasmania.

CHARACTERISTICS:
Eucalyptus blue gum, also known as Tasmanian blue gum, is a clear or colorless thin oil that easily drops from the bottle dropper.

FRAGRANCE DESCRIPTION:
Eucalyptus has fresh, sharp, camphoraceous top notes with intense, woody, penetrating, undertones.

SAFE USAGE: Use carefully in small amounts, but all the eucalyptus varieties are safe when used correctly for external applications. Although it is recommended never to ingest any essential oil internally, eucalyptus is very toxic if swallowed so make sure to keep the bottle well away from children.

PLANT DESCRIPTION

There are over 600 species of eucalyptus, of which about 20 are used to produce essential oils. Eucalyptus are tall, fast-growing evergreen trees with long, narrow leaves, and white-yellow flowers. As well as the traditional *globulus* (or blue gum), *citriodora* (or lemon-scented), *radiata* (or narrow-leaved), *dives* (or broad-leaved peppermint), *polybractea* and *smithii* (or gully gum), are the main species used in aromatherapy.

BLENDING PROFILE

In small amounts, eucalyptus blends well with most other wood and herbal oils, and also with lavender and lemon.

TRADITIONAL USES

The timber of eucalyptus is used in construction and building. In World War I eucalyptus oil was used to treat meningitis and flu. The oil can be used to remove tar and oil from the skin. Eucalyptus oil is used extensively in medical remedies for inhalations, lozenges, rubs, and gargles, and it is perhaps the most familiar of essential oils to the general public.

With the recent introduction of other species, blue gum is less used than it used to be as it is quite harsh, while *citriodora*, *radiata*, and *smithii* are gentler, especially in inhalations.

THERAPEUTIC PROPERTIES

Analgesic, antibacterial, antineuralgic, antiseptic, antirheumatic, antispasmodic, antiviral, astringent, balsamic, decongestant, deodorant, diuretic, expectorant, febrifuge, rubefacient, vermifuge, and vulnerary. *(See glossary on page 158.)*

Relieves colds

Eucalyptus is probably the most commonly used essential oil. It is widely used as a decongestant in steam inhalations to relieve colds, flu, and other respiratory ailments. Sniffed from a tissue, blue gum clears the head wonderfully and relieves headaches and neuralgia. It is also indicated in massage, in small amounts, to relieve muscular aches and pains. Blue gum helps alleviate urinary tract infections. An interesting use of blue gum is removing tar or oil stains from feet, if your holiday beach has tar deposits. Overall, blue gum eucalyptus is stimulating, refreshing, and clearing.

Refreshing and pain-relieving

Eucalyptus radiata used in the bath or a local wash helps relieve the pain of shingles, and when blended with bergamot it is effective against herpes, including cold sores. Both *radiata* and *smithii* are better than blue gum in steam inhalations for colds, phlegm, sinusitis, and other respiratory ailments, as they are gentler and better tolerated.

Citriodora is an excellent choice to use with colds, sore throats, and flu. In steam inhalations, it clears the sinuses and relieves headaches, and in the bath, lemon eucalyptus is refreshing and uplifting. *Citriodora* is also good for athlete's foot, herpes, and dandruff. It is an excellent insect repellant and its analgesic properties make it effective for pain relief in the treatment of bites and stings.

Stimulating and purifying

Psychologically, eucalyptus is piercing, stimulating, and purifying. It is useful in meditation when you have a cold to help keep the mind clear. Eucalyptus is a tonic of subtle energy, especially of the lungs, and helps those who feel constricted in their lives. It can be used in a burner as a psychic cleanser, to rid rooms of negative energy.

Insect repellent spray

This spray is especially effective against mosquitoes. The citronella brings a refreshing lemon note to the more pungent eucalyptus. Use the spray on your body, clothes, and bedding. Apply onto areas of bare skin (except the face) and spray your room and bedding at night when mosquitoes are likely to be active. Reapply as necessary.

You will need:

- 1 x 3½ fl oz (100 ml) dark glass spray bottle
- 1 tsp perfumer's alcohol (see page 40)

- 20 drops eucalyptus blue gum essential oil
- 20 drops citronella essential oil
- 3 fl oz (90 ml) witch hazel

1. Measure the perfumer's alcohol into a glass jug. Add the essential oils and stir well to thoroughly dissolve.

2. Pour into the bottle, top up with witch hazel, and shake gently. Label the bottle with ingredients, amounts, and the date.

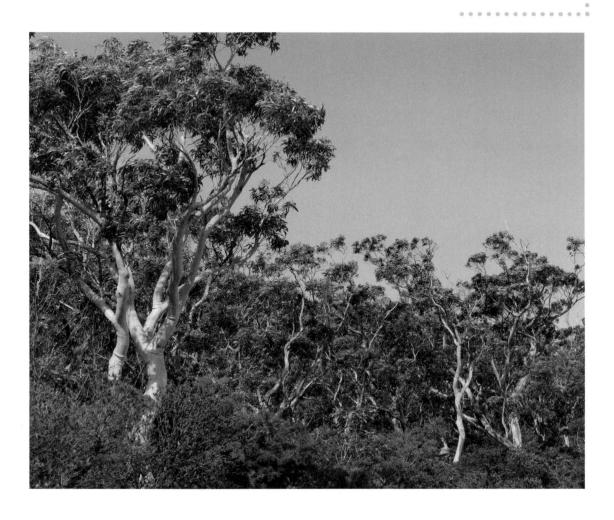

PINE NEEDLES

Pinus sylvestris

Botanical Family:
Pinaceae

Traditional uses of pine include bathing with young shoots in the water to alleviate a wide range of conditions, including nervous exhaustion, painful joints, and skin problems.

METHOD OF EXTRACTION:
Pine needles essential oil is sometimes steam distilled from the needles, young branches, and cones. The best for aromatherapy use is dry distillation of the needles only.

REGIONS OF ORIGIN:
Americas, Austria, Finland, Hungary, Russia.

CHARACTERISTICS:
Pine needles is a clear thin oil that easily drops from the bottle dropper.

FRAGRANCE DESCRIPTION:
Pine needles has fresh, turpentine, coniferous, camphoraceous top notes with dry, sweet, balsamic, woody undertones.

SAFE USAGE: Do not use if you have sensitive skin, asthma, or kidney disease. Use carefully in small amounts.

PLANT DESCRIPTION

Pine is also known as Scots pine and Norway pine. It is a tall evergreen tree growing to over 115 feet in height at maturity, with distinctive fissured, reddish-brown bark, pine needles, and pine cones. There are many different varieties of pine, some of which are also used to produce essential oil. However, Scots pine is the safest and best to use therapeutically.

BLENDING PROFILE

Pine needles blends well with most other wood and herbal oils, also lavender and lemon.

TRADITIONAL USES

Native Americans used pine needles in their bedding to repel insects. Pine needles oil is much used in pharmaceutical preparations for coughs, colds, decongestants, and analgesic ointments. The aromatherapy pioneer Marguerite Maury used pine needles essential oil to treat rheumatic conditions, as a diuretic, and to help treat pulmonary infections. Pine needles is used in air fresheners, domestic cleaners, and detergents.

THERAPEUTIC PROPERTIES

Antimicrobial, antineuralgic, antiseptic, antirheumatic, antiviral, balsamic, bactericidal, cholagogue, deodorant, diuretic, expectorant, insecticide, rubefacient, and tonic. *(See glossary on page 158.)*

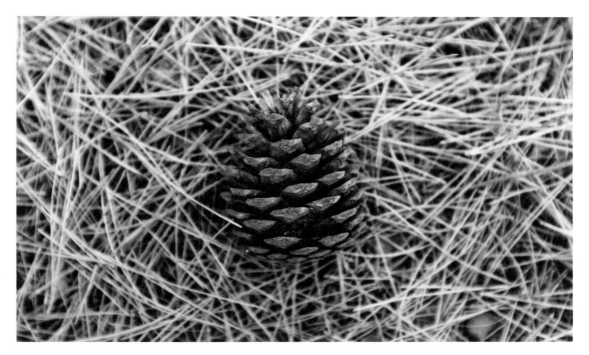

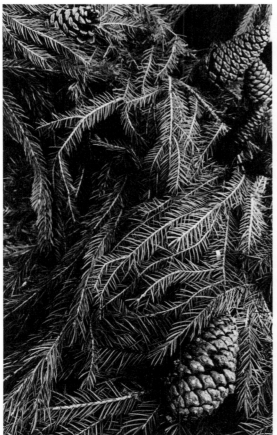

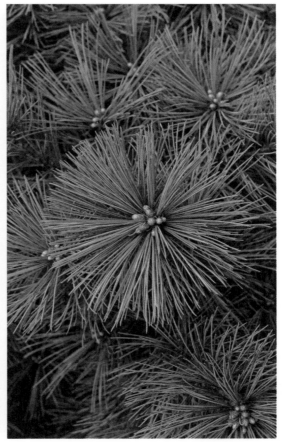

Restorative and strengthening

The best quality pine needles essential oil comes from the Austrian Tyrol. Pine needles is an excellent expectorant and is indicated for all respiratory complaints. It is among the best choices to clear phlegm from the lungs, and is good for sinusitis and all bronchial conditions. Pine needles is a tonic of the lungs, kidneys, and nervous system, and is also considered an adrenal stimulant. Its clear, piercing properties makes pine needles effective in relieving fatigue and nervous exhaustion, and it is also helpful for general debility and in convalescence. Overall, pine needles is restorative, reviving, and strengthening.

Its stimulating and analgesic properties make pine needles a good choice to use in compresses and massage after long periods of exercise, and for sports injuries. It also helps with painful joints in a hot compress. Pine needles can help with cystitis and other urinary complaints, especially if the kidneys are weak.

Instills self-confidence

Psychologically, pine needles is warming and cleansing. It tones subtle energy, and is good burned before meditations to psychically cleanse the space. Pine needles instills self-confidence and allays guilt, helping bring about acceptance and forgiveness. As a symbol of endurance, the will to survive, and being a free spirit, pine needles encourages perseverance, courage, and patience.

Natural floor cleaner

Washing your floors with this natural, homemade, pine-scented cleaner is a great way to be actively eco-conscious. Chemical cleaning products are linked evermore frequently to increased incidents of asthma, eczema, allergies, cancer, and other illnesses, as well as causing headaches. With shop-bought cleaners, there is also the possibility of accidental poisoning, as most contain toxic ingredients. These natural ingredients and essential oils give your house a clean, fresh scent, as well as getting rid of dirt, germs, and bacteria. The pine needles and lemon oil help boost your immune system and their natural scent will lift your mood.

You will need:

- a bucket
- 1 tsp soda crystals or bicarbonate of soda
- splash of white vinegar
- 10 drops pine needles essential oil
- 5 drops lemon essential oil

1. Half fill the bucket with hot water.

2. Add the soda crystals or bicarbonate of soda and stir well to dissolve.

3. Add a splash of white vinegar and the essential oils. Slosh around the liquid in the bucket to mix everything thoroughly.

4. Use as you would your regular cleaner on ceramic tiles, vinyl, laminate, and hardwood floors.

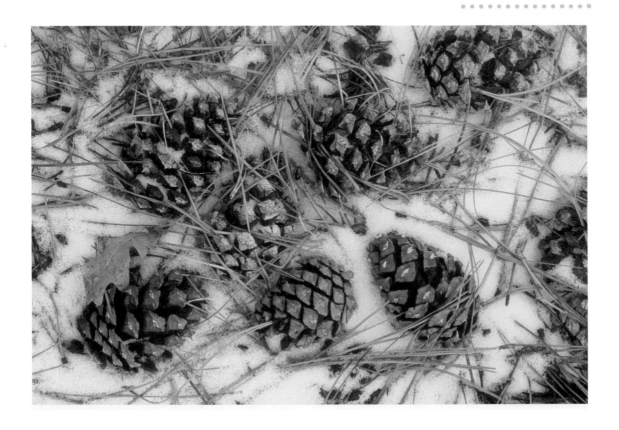

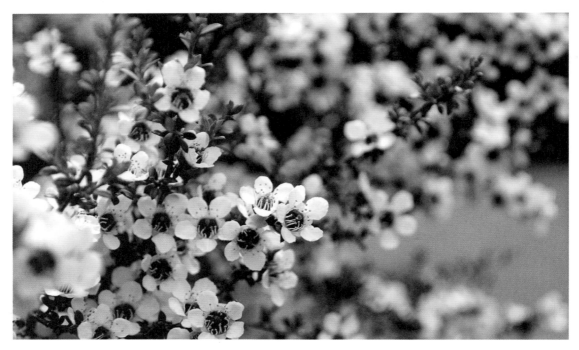

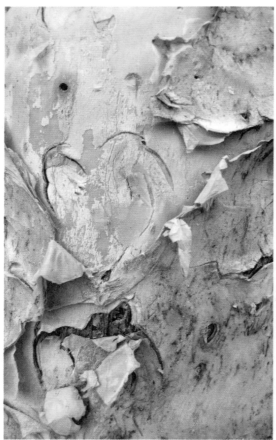

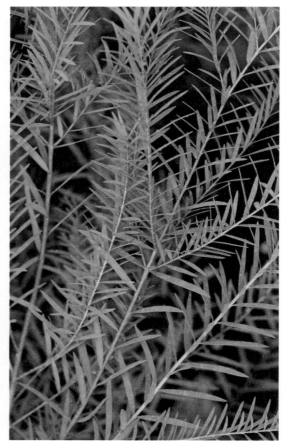

TEA TREE

Melaleuca alternifolia

Botanical Family:
Myrtaceae

Tea tree has long been used by indigenous Australian people, often by simply crushing leaves in the hand and inhaling the volatile oils to relieve headaches, colds, and congestion.

METHOD OF EXTRACTION:
Tea tree essential oil is steam or water distilled from the leaves and twigs.

REGIONS OF ORIGIN:
Australia.

CHARACTERISTICS:
Tea tree is a clear thin oil that easily drops from the bottle dropper.

FRAGRANCE DESCRIPTION:
Tea tree has warm, spicy, camphoraceous top notes with pungent, medicinal undertones.

SAFE USAGE: Do not use on very sensitive skin. Use in moderation: No more than 3 drops in the bath, and no more than 2% dilution in massage oils. Avoid direct contact with the skin, except directly on spots, veruccas, and cold sores.

PLANT DESCRIPTION

Tea tree is a small shrub-like tree reaching over 20 feet at maturity, with off-white flowers, and needle-like leaves. It grows best in swampy ground in subtropical conditions. Also known as paper bark, the bark of tea tree is white and papery.

BLENDING PROFILE

Tea tree in small amounts blends well with most spice and herbal oils, also lavender, pine needles, bergamot, and eucalyptus.

TRADITIONAL USES

Captain Cook first coined the name of tea tree in 1777 when the leaves were steeped in water and the resulting "tea" drunk to prevent scurvy. The oil was first distilled in the 1920s and was one of the first essential oils to be exported, and widely sold and used in Europe.

THERAPEUTIC PROPERTIES

Antimicrobial, antifungal, antiseptic, antiviral, bactericide, cicatrisant, expectorant, fungicide, immunostimulant, insecticide, stimulant, and sudorific. *(See glossary on page 158.)*

A powerful healer
Tea tree is the most "medicinal" of the essential oils, with powerful antimicrobial activity against all three

of the infectious organisms: Bacteria, viruses and fungi. The *Melaleuca* family also includes niaouli (*Melaleuca quinquenervia*), which is similar to tea tree but is gentler and better tolerated on the skin, making it a useful and sweeter-smelling alternative. When diffused in a burner, tea tree helps prevent the spread of infection. Together with its powerful immunostimulant properties, tea tree helps combat many illnesses and ailments. Overall, tea tree is penetrating, medicinal, and stimulating.

Athlete's foot, vaginal thrush, herpes infections (including cold sores), insect bites, spots, acne, and minor abrasions all respond well to local applications of tea tree, either diluted, or a drop applied carefully so as not to damage the surrounding skin. Tea tree is effective because it is strong and needs to be treated with respect. For washing abrasions or a local wash for vaginal thrush, dilute 2 drops in a little perfumer's alcohol and mix with 2 fl oz (50 ml) of water; this low dilution is safe yet still effective. For spots and cold sores, use a cottonwool bud with 1 drop of tea tree and apply carefully to the affected area, avoiding the surrounding skin.

Boosts immune system

In steam inhalations tea tree prevents colds and flu developing: If they do manifest, it aids recovery and alleviates symptoms. It also helps clear coughs, sinusitis, bronchitis, and other respiratory conditions. Tea tree in massage and bath oils can boost a weak immune system, and it helps with long-term debilitating illnesses, such as glandular fever. Mixed into aloe vera gel, tea tree helps alleviate the pain of shingles.

Psychologically, tea tree is strengthening and warming. The aroma of tea tree is distinctly medicinal and many people find it more palatable when blended. Tea tree invigorates mind, body, and spirit; it inspires confidence and dispels the gloom of chronic ill health. Tea tree also strengthens subtle energies.

Tea tree first-aid gel

The best way to use tea tree safely but effectively, and avoid any risk of damaging the skin, is to dilute it. One of the most useful mediums for this is aloe vera gel, which is easily available from natural health and aromatherapy websites. Aloe vera gel is made from the fleshy parts of the aloe vera plant and renowned for its healing properties.

You will need:

- 1 small glass jar
- 2 tsp aloe vera gel
- 4 drops tea tree essential oil

1. Carefully spoon the aloe vera gel into the jar, drip in the tea tree oil and use a chopstick or glass stirring rod to mix the ingredients together well.

2. Label the jar with the ingredients, amounts, and date.

3. Use this healing gel on spots, cuts and grazes, shingles, and athlete's foot. Reapply as required.

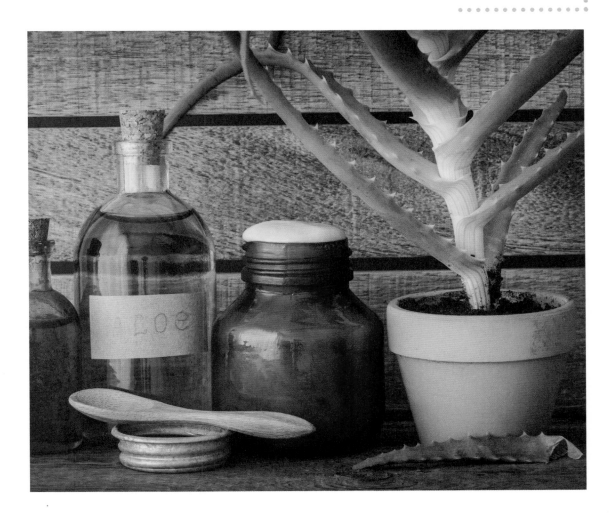

CEDARWOOD ATLAS

Cedrus atlantica

Botanical Family:
Pinaceae

Cedarwood atlas essential oil was traditionally used to treat bronchial and urinary tract infections, and also as a preservative and in incense.

METHOD OF EXTRACTION:
Cedarwood atlas essential oil is steam distilled from wood chips, preferably from the heart wood.

REGIONS OF ORIGIN:
Algeria, Cyprus, Lebanon, Morocco.

CHARACTERISTICS:
Cedarwood atlas is a viscous oil that with a little patience easily drops from the bottle dropper.

FRAGRANCE DESCRIPTION:
Cedarwood has turpentine, woody, camphor-like top notes with deep, sweet, balsamic, smoky undertones.

SAFE USAGE: Avoid during pregnancy.

PLANT DESCRIPTION

The modern-day cedarwood atlas originated from the famous biblical cedars of Lebanon, where they grew freely and abundantly. Cedarwood atlas trees also grew wild in Cyprus. The word *cedrus* originates from the Arabic *kedron*, which means power. Cedarwood atlas is a tall, majestic evergreen tree that grows to over 100 feet at maturity and lives for over 1,000 years. It's important to make sure the essential oil you purchase is cedarwood atlas. There is also frequently available cedarwood Virginian, but this essential oil needs to be used carefully and is therefore not recommended for general use.

BLENDING PROFILE

Cedarwood atlas blends well with most other wood oils, and also with jasmine, black pepper, cardamom, frankincense, vetivert, patchouli, rosemary, lemon, sweet orange, and bergamot.

TRADITIONAL USES

In the Bible, the Song of Solomon tells us that his famous temple was built from cedarwood, and that the building symbolized the abundance, dignity, and strength displayed by the cedarwood tree. The original Lebanese cedars may have produced the first essential oil that was used by the ancient Egyptians for embalming bodies, and in perfumery and cosmetics.

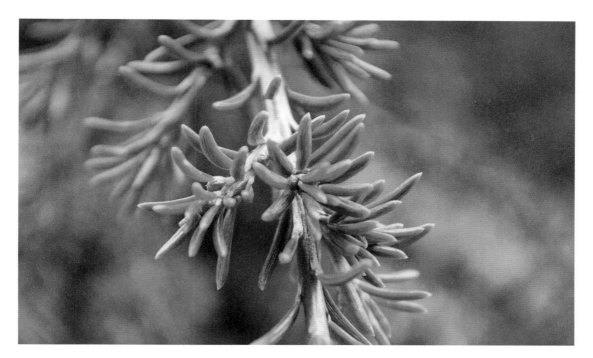

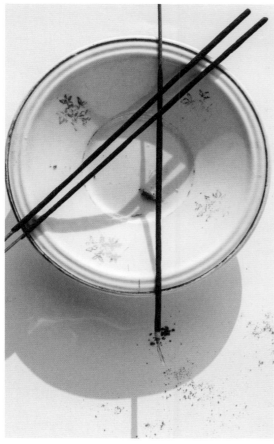

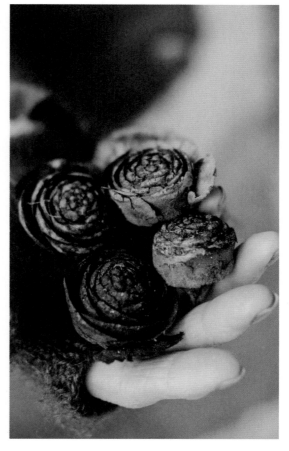

Cedarwood was an ingredient in *mithridate*, a much-valued antidote to poison with a long history of use. Cedarwood trees were valued for their wood because buildings and furniture would be safe from harmful insects, as the highly fragrant wood repelled them. The Tibetans still use cedarwood atlas in their medicine and incense.

THERAPEUTIC PROPERTIES

Antiseptic, astringent, antiseborrheic, diuretic, expectorant, insecticide, and sedative.
(See glossary on page 158.)

Masculine fragrance

Cedarwood atlas is the first choice for men's skin and haircare products because of its familiar masculine fragrance. Mixed into base creams, lotions, and toners, cedarwood atlas improves oily skin and acne, while mixed into base shampoo and conditioner, it tones the scalp and helps prevent dandruff.

Treats coughs and bronchitis

In local, full-body massage and hot compresses, cedarwood atlas is useful for treating urinary tract infections, while in steam inhalations and burners, it is recommended for coughs and chronic bronchitis. It has a mild diuretic action and is a useful alternative in lymphatic massage blends to help reduce cellulite and edema. Overall, cedarwood atlas is fortifying, calming, and opening.

Instills courage

Psychologically, cedarwood atlas reduces fear and helps you discover inner strength and courage. It is good for calming nervous tension and stress, particularly when mixed into blends used for full body massage, and is welcomed by those who prefer a masculine fragrance. Cedarwood atlas is good in meditations, especially helping instill confidence, and it is an effective general tonic for strengthening subtle energies.

Cedarwood atlas aftershave

This homemade cedarwood atlas aftershave will be much appreciated for its skin toning, refreshing, and tightening qualities on the face after shaving as well as for its natural masculine scent.

You will need:

- 1 x 3½ fl oz (100 ml) dark glass bottle
- 1 tsp perfumer's alcohol (see page 40)
- 8 drops cedarwood atlas essential oil
- 4 drops vetivert essential oil
- 2 drops juniper berry essential oil (substitute bergamot for sensitive skin)
- 3½ fl oz (100 ml) witch hazel
- 3½ fl oz (100 ml) orange flower water for (sensitive skins substitute with rose water)

1. Measure the perfumer's alcohol and pour into the bottle.

2. Carefully drip out the required number of drops of cedarwood, vetivert, and juniper berry into the bottle and shake well to dissolve the oils in the alcohol.

3. Top up with witch hazel and orange flower water and shake again.

4. Label the bottle with the ingredients, amounts used, and date.

5. The cedarwood aftershave can be splashed on the face in the same way as shop-bought aftershave.

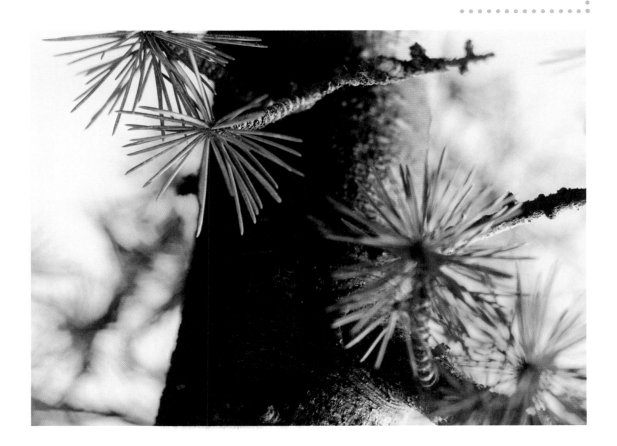

GINGER

Zingiber officinale

Botanical Family:
Zingiberaceae

A familiar culinary spice, ginger is warming and stimulating. It is excellent used in winter to physically and psychologically fortify the body and emotions.

METHOD OF EXTRACTION:
The essential oil is steam distilled from the unpeeled, dried, ground rhizome.

REGIONS OF ORIGIN:
Australia, China, India, Japan, Southeast Asia, Thailand.

CHARACTERISTICS:
Ginger is a pale yellow or orange thin oil that easily drops from the bottle dropper. Ginger essential oil becomes viscous with age.

FRAGRANCE DESCRIPTION:
Giner has sharp, green top notes and fiery, woody, warm, rich, sweet, spicy undertones.

SAFE USAGE: Do not use if you have very sensitive skin. Use no more than 3 drops in the bath, and use no more than 2% dilution in massage oils.

PLANT DESCRIPTION

Ginger is a perennial, tropical plant with reed-like leaves, white, purple or yellow flowers, and a thick tuberous rhizome near the surface of the soil.

BLENDING PROFILE

Ginger blends well with other spice oils and citrus oils, and also with sweet marjoram, sweet fennel, clary sage, neroli, geranium, ylang ylang, rose, jasmine, lavender, lemongrass, frankincense, sandalwood, vetivert, patchouli, and petitgrain.

TRADITIONAL USES

Ginger was mentioned in the earliest Sanskrit texts. It was used in ancient India as a spice, and also medicinally, and it is still used in Ayurvedic medicine. Ginger was also used in ancient China and Middle Eastern cultures. In Traditional Chinese Medicine, ginger is used to alleviate colds and chills, promote sweating, and stimulate the appetite. Infusions of ginger were used to treat stomach and digestive disorders, nausea, cholera, and bleeding.

Exported along the Spice Route, ginger was introduced to the New World by the Portuguese. The ancient Greeks and Romans also used ginger. It is a familiar culinary spice, and is also eaten as stem ginger and crystallized ginger. There are a variety of ginger teas.

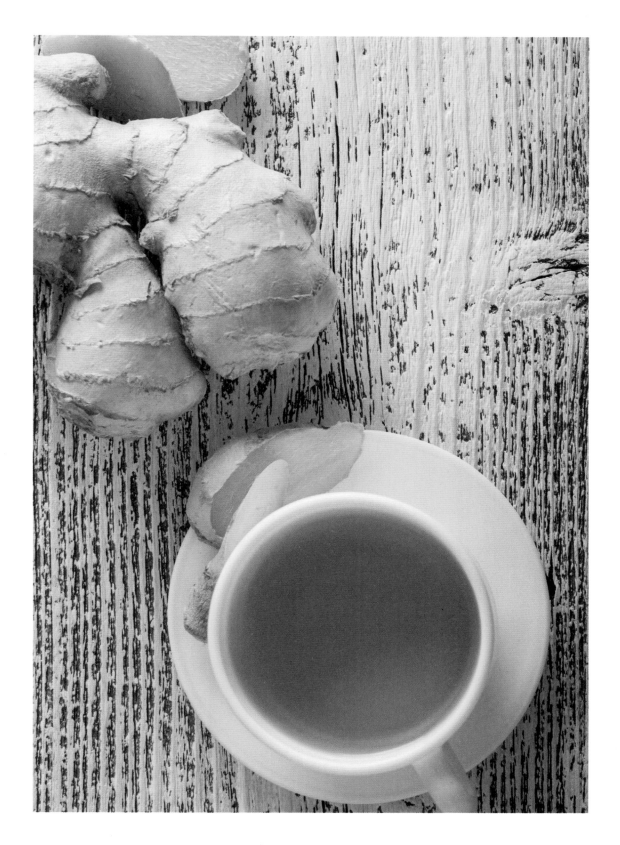

THERAPEUTIC PROPERTIES

Aanalgesic, antiseptic, aphrodisiac, bactericide, carminative, cephalic, digestive, expectorant, febrifuge, laxative, rubefacient, stimulant, sudorific, and tonic. *(See glossary on page 158.)*

Stimulating and tonic

Ginger is warming and stimulates circulation and digestion. It is a tonic for the heart, and is indicated in baths and massage for poor circulation, cardiac fatigue, and for cold hands and feet. It is useful for respiratory complaints, as it is a bronchodilator and helps open congested airways. Overall, ginger is warming, comforting, and fortifying.

Improves digestion

Its stimulant properties make ginger useful for flatulence and poor digestion. When sniffed from a tissue, blended into a perfume, or drunk as a tea, it is useful for travel sickness, morning sickness, and other nausea and vomiting. Ginger is good in massage when the muscles are tired and aching, particularly when they are cold and contracted. Ginger can be useful in a bath or inhalation when you have a cold, cough, or sore throat, as its sharp, piercing fragrance cuts through catarrh and congestion. Ginger is also good in massage blends, to warm and relieve painful, overworked muscles.

Inspires initiative

Psychologically, ginger is arousing, opulent, and stimulating. It is indicated for use in meditation when there is debility through nervous exhaustion. Ginger warms and strengthens the emotions, increases determination, and inspires initiative and action to carry plans through to their conclusion. Ginger helps dispel the winter blues and is useful in combating Seasonal Affective Disorder, especially when blended with bergamot.

Ginger loaf cake

This sticky, treacly cake is a wonderful way to enjoy the benefits of ginger.

You will need:

- 2 cups all-purpose flour
- 1 tsp mixed spice
- 2 tsp ground ginger
- 1½ tsp baking powder
- ½ tsp bicarbonate of soda
- ½ tsp salt
- 1¼ cups milk
- 1 egg
- ¾ stick butter
- ¼ cup black treacle
- ¼ cup golden syrup
- ½ cup superfine sugar
- 6 drops ginger essential oil

1. Heat the oven to 350°F/180°C. Lightly grease a 2 lb (900 g) loaf tin and line with baking parchment.

2. Sift the flour, mixed spice, ground ginger, baking power, bicarbonate of soda, and salt into a large mixing bowl.

3. Pour the milk into a jug and beat in the egg.

4. Place the butter, treacle, golden syrup, and sugar in a pan and heat gently, stirring occasionally, until the butter has melted. Add the essential oil and remove immediately from the heat.

5. Pour the butter and sugar mixture into the dry ingredients, followed by the milk and egg mixture, and beat with a wooden spoon until all the ingredients are well mixed.

6. Pour the batter into the loaf tin and bake for 90 minutes, or until the cake feels firm and a skewer inserted into the middle comes out clean. Leave in its tin until cool enough to handle, then turn out onto a wire rack.

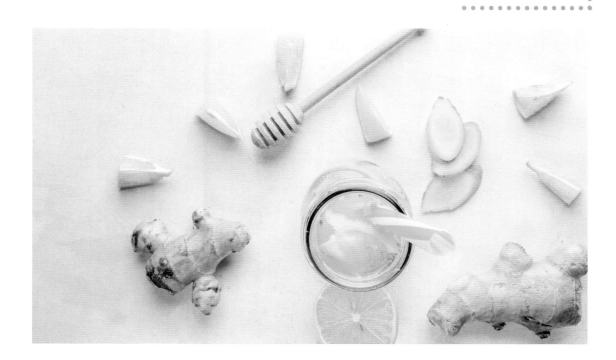

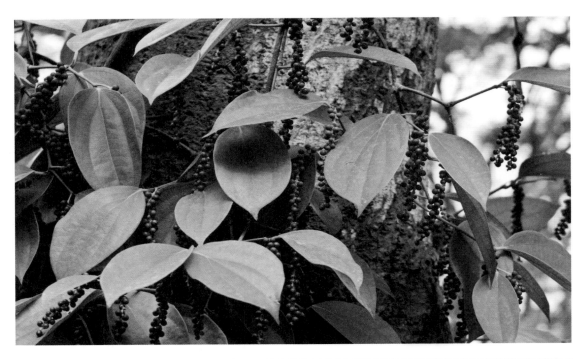

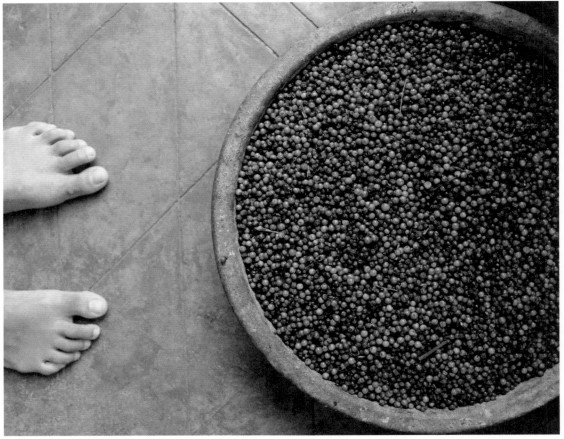

BLACK PEPPER

Piper nigrum L.

Botanical Family:
Piperaceae

Psychologically, black pepper is warming, builds endurance, and helps you reconnect with life whenever you feel alienated.

METHOD OF EXTRACTION:
The essential oil is steam distilled from the dried, crushed almost ripe berries.

REGIONS OF ORIGIN:
India, Indonesia, Madagascar.

CHARACTERISTICS:
Black pepper is a clear or pale green thin essential oil that drops easily from the bottle dropper.

FRAGRANCE DESCRIPTION:
Black pepper has hot, spicy, fiery top notes with warm, sharp, dry woody, oriental undertones.

SAFE USAGE: Do not use if you have very sensitive skin. Use no more than 3 drops in the bath, and use no more than 2% dilution in massage oils.

PLANT DESCRIPTION

Black pepper originated in the hills of western India. It is a perennial, woody vine with heart-shaped shiny leaves, and yellow-green or white flowers, which turn into berries, also called peppercorns.

BLENDING PROFILE

In small amounts black pepper blends well with the other spice oils and most floral oils, as well as frankincense, sandalwood, cedarwood atlas, sweet marjoram, clary sage, sweet basil, sweet fennel, lemongrass, eucalyptus, and rosemary.

TRADITIONAL USES

Black pepper has been esteemed as a spice and valuable trading commodity since antiquity. The name derives from the Sanskrit *pippali*. In ancient Greece and Europe during the Middle Ages, it was used to season and preserve meats. Herbalists used it to treat digestive complaints. Some Chinese monks would swallow one peppercorn a day, which they believed gave endurance, allowing them to travel vast distances.

Black pepper is still widely used as a culinary spice, and in Traditional Chinese Medicine, and Indian Ayurvedic medicine.

THERAPEUTIC PROPERTIES

Analgesic, anticatarrhal, antiseptic, antispasmodic, aphrodisiac, bactericide, carminative, diaphoretic, digestive, expectorant, febrifuge, laxative, rubefacient, stimulant, stomachic, and tonic. *(See glossary on page 158.)*

Digestive stimulant

Black pepper is an excellent stimulant for the digestive system. When blended with sweet marjoram and sweet orange and used in firm abdominal massage, black pepper helps to alleviate constipation. It also stimulates the appetite and helps relieve flatulence, colic, loss of appetite, and nausea. It stimulates the spleen, so it is useful in treating anemia. Black pepper can be used in compresses to treat bruises and chilblains.

Fortifying and stimulating

Black pepper essential oil is useful in massage to stimulate and warm tight muscles and to relieve rheumatism, arthritis, and all forms of joint or muscle pain. It is also indicated for colds, flu, and minor infections. For these conditions, it is best used in a low dilution in a bath, together with lavender, frankincense, ravintsara, eucalyptus, or tea tree. Overall, black pepper is fortifying, strengthening, and stimulating.

Mystery and intrigue

Black pepper is full of mystery and intrigue, and fortifies mind and spirit. Its slight aphrodisiac quality is especially useful for those whose sensual emotions lack fire and passion. Black pepper is indicated in meditation when you feel cold and aloof, and it helps you move on when you feel stuck and trapped.

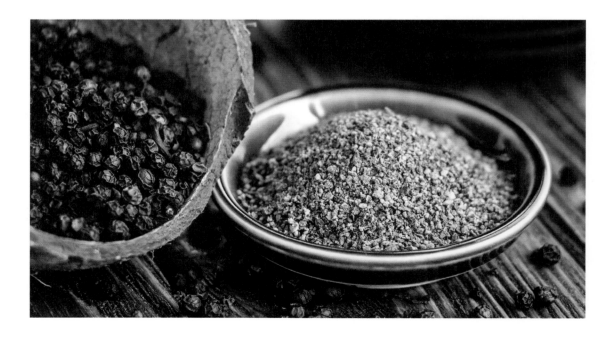

Black pepper tofu

Make this delicious dish in colder months to help fight off winter ailments. Black pepper tofu is nutritious and vegetarian.

You will need:

For the marinade:
- 3 garlic cloves, crushed
- 2 tsp soy sauce
- 1 tsp brown sugar
- 3 tbsp groundnut oil
- 1 tbsp sesame oil
- 6 drops black pepper essential oil

For the tofu:
- 1 packet firm tofu, cut into medium-sized slices
- 6 tbsp groundnut oil
- ½ cup vegetable stock
- 2 tbsp soy sauce
- 1 tsp sundried tomato purée
- 1 tbsp rice vinegar
- 1 tsp cornstarch or arrowroot
- 1 tsp coarsely ground black pepper
- 2 tsp sesame oil

To garnish:
- coriander leaves, finely chopped
- ½ cucumber, thinly sliced
- 2 spring onions, thinly sliced

1. Mix the marinade ingredients together in a small bowl and stir well until the sugar is dissolved.

2. Place the tofu in a large, flat dish and pour over the marinade. Leave for 30 minutes to 1 hour.

3. Heat the groundnut oil and fry the tofu until golden brown on both sides. Remove from the pan and place on kitchen paper to absorb excess oil.

4. Wipe the pan clean, then pour in the vegetable stock, soy sauce, tomato purée, and rice vinegar. Add a little water to the cornstarch or arrowroot to make a paste and add to the pan, stirring. Bring to a boil, stirring, until the mixture thickens. Add the tofu and heat through.

5. Remove the pan from the heat and stir in the black pepper and sesame oil. Transfer to a serving dish and sprinkle over the garnishes.

CARDAMOM

Ellettaria cardamomum

Botanical Family:
Zingiberaceae

The word cardamom probably originated from the Arab word *hehmama,* a derivation from Sanskrit, meaning hot and pungent.

METHOD OF EXTRACTION:
Cardamom essential oil
is steam distilled from
the dried, ripe seeds, or
sometimes from the fresh
seeds. A CO_2 extraction is
occasionally available.

REGIONS OF ORIGIN:
Guatemala, India, Sri Lanka.

CHARACTERISTICS:
Cardamom is a clear or pale
yellow, thin essential oil that
easily drops from the bottle
dropper. It colors when
exposed to sunlight, so store
in the dark.

FRAGRANCE DESCRIPTION:
Cardamom has warm,
sweet, spicy top notes
with woody, balsamic,
camphoraceous undertones.

SAFE USAGE: Do not use if you have
very sensitive skin. Use no more than
3 drops in the bath, and use no more
than 2% dilution in massage oils.

PLANT DESCRIPTION

Cardamom is a perennial, reed-like plant growing out
of a rhizome. The plant has long, blade-shaped leaves,
and pale green or yellow flowers (sometimes with
purple tips), which are later followed by oblong
red-brown or green seed pods.

BLENDING PROFILE

Cardamom blends well with most other spice oils,
citrus and floral oils, as well as frankincense, sandalwood,
vetivert, patchouli, cedarwood atlas, sweet fennel, sweet
marjoram, clary sage, and rosemary.

TRADITIONAL USES

Reputed to be one of the oldest spices, cardamom
was referred to on an ancient Sumatran clay tablet.
Cardamom has been used for centuries in Chinese
and Ayurvedic medicine for all digestive complaints.
According to an ancient Vedic text, cardamom is reputed
to be an aphrodisiac, although its potency in this area is
best brought out by blending with other aphrodisiac oils.

Cardamom was traditionally used in incense by both
Hindu and Tibetan cultures and has a long history of
being used in perfumery. The Greeks brought cardamom
to Europe in the 4th century BCE. The whole seed pods
and the ground powder remain an important culinary
spice worldwide.

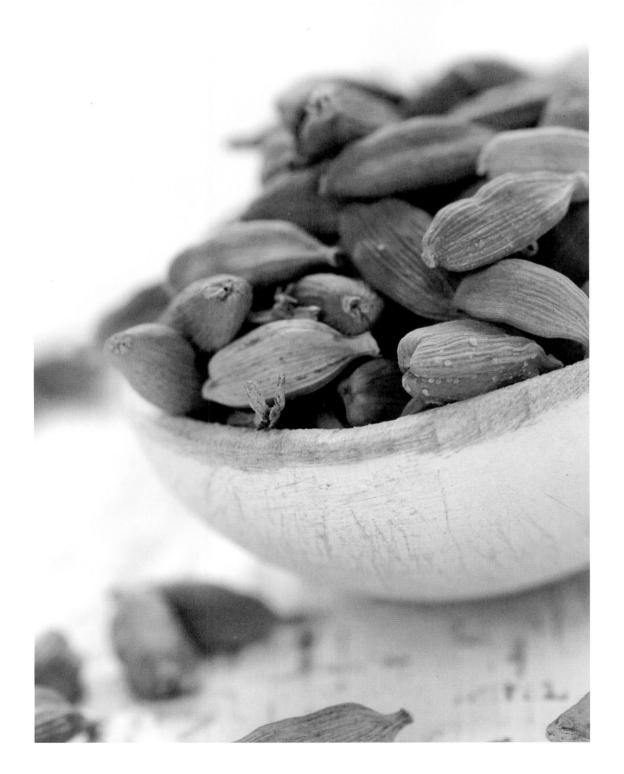

THERAPEUTIC PROPERTIES

Antiseptic, antispasmodic, carminative, cephalic, digestive, diuretic, expectorant, rubefacient, stimulant, stomachic, and tonic. *(See glossary on page 158.)*

Excellent tonic

Cardamom is one of the best tonic essential oils. As well as having a general and overall tonic effect on the body, cardamom is an effective tonic of the nerves and of the subtle energies. It is indicated for both digestive and respiratory problems, particularly those of a damp origin or nature, such as flatulence, chronic bronchitis, and colic. For these conditions cardamom is best used in local massage and in the bath. Cardamom also helps with cramp, dyspepsia, and indigestion. Overall, cardamom is warming, gentle, and penetrating.

Lifts the spirits

Psychologically, cardamom is fortifying, and uplifting, and good for nervous exhaustion and mental fatigue. For psychological and emotional conditions, cardamom is best blended into a perfume, along with other appropriate essential oils, especially floral and citrus oils, such as rose and mandarin.

Cardamom fortifies those who feel overburdened with cares, worries, and responsibilities; it lifts the spirits and inspires courage and fortitude. It is associated with the Earth element, and is grounding for those who tend to feel "spaced out."

Masala chai tea

This traditional chai recipe uses several spices as well as cardamom, but it is the cardamom that gives the unique flavor to the drink. Chai is a ubiquitous spiced Indian tea. The "chai wallah" is a familiar sight on Indian streets, bus stations, and train platforms and makes each little cup of chai freshly—and, of course, each chai wallah has their own special blend. For this recipe you can use already ground spices for convenience but freshly ground spices are better.

You will need:

- 1 heaped tbsp small-leafed tea (such as Assam)
- 1-in (2½-cm) piece ginger, chopped
- 1 tsp cinnamon
- 1 tsp nutmeg
- 1 tsp black pepper
- 1 tsp clove
- 1 tsp cardamom
- ½ cup milk
- 1 tsp sugar

1. Boil ½ cup water in a small pan. Add the tea, chopped fresh ginger, and ground spices. You can substitute 1 drop of essential oil for any of the spices.

2. Boil for 1–2 minutes, then add the milk and sugar and bring to the boil again.

3. Strain into a cup and drink hot.

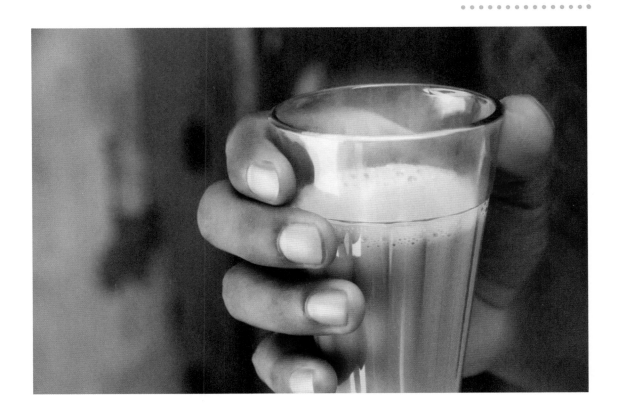

CINNAMON LEAF

Cinnamomum zeylanicum

Botanical Family:
Lauraceae

Cinnamon leaf has a long tradition of use for respiratory infections, digestive complaints, menstruation problems, rheumatism, tight muscles, and as a stimulant.

METHOD OF EXTRACTION:
Cinnamon essential oil is steam or water distilled from the leaves and small twigs.

REGIONS OF ORIGIN:
Africa, Burma, Comoros Islands, Jamaica, Madagascar, South India, Southeast Asia, Sri Lanka.

CHARACTERISTICS:
Cinnamon leaf is a pale yellow or brown thin essential oil that drops easily from the bottle dropper.

FRAGRANCE DESCRIPTION:
Cinnamon leaf has fiery, warm, spicy top notes and sweet, oriental undertones.

SAFE USAGE: Do not use if you have sensitive skin. Use in moderation; no more than 2 drops in the bath.

PLANT DESCRIPTION

Cinnamon is an evergreen tree growing up to 50 feet.

BLENDING PROFILE

Cinnamon leaf blends well with other spice and citrus oils, as well as lavender, frankincense, myrrh, benzoin, lemongrass, palmarosa, and ylang ylang.

TRADITIONAL USES

Cinnamon leaf is used in toiletries, perfumes, toothpaste, mouthwash, and culinary flavorings.

THERAPEUTIC PROPERTIES

Antiseptic, antispasmodic, antimicrobial, astringent, carminative, digestive, emmenagogue, stimulant, stomachic, and vermifuge. *(See glossary on page 158.)*

When diffused in a burner, cinnamon leaf wards off colds and flu. Blended into massage oil with sweet orange and sweet marjoram, cinnamon leaf is good for digestive complaints, flatulence, and intestinal infections. Useful in massage for sluggish circulation, joint pain, and overworked muscles, cinnamon leaf is also an aphrodisiac. Blended with floral and citrus oils in a sensuous massage between lovers, it can be used to "spice up" a flagging libido. Overall, cinnamon leaf is warming, restorative, and uplifting.

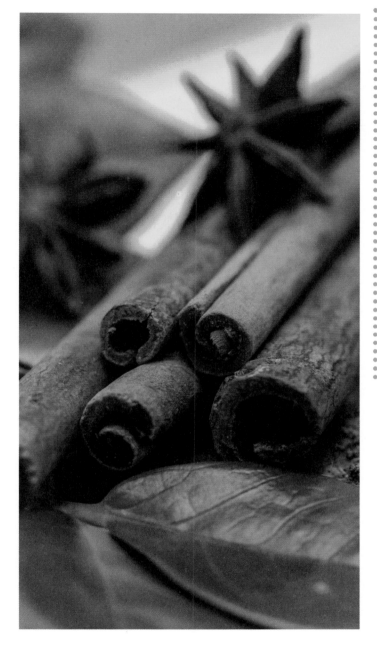

Cinnamon bran muffins

These tasty muffins stimulate a sluggish digestion.

You will need:

- 2 eggs
- ¾ cup brown sugar
- 2 bananas, mashed
- 1¼ cups buttermilk
- 3½ cups wheat or oat bran
- 2 tbsp rapeseed oil
- 1 tsp vanilla essence
- 4 drops cinnamon leaf essential oil
- 1¾ cups whole wheat flour
- 1½ cups all-purpose flour
- 1½ tsp baking powder
- ½ tsp bicarbonate of soda
- ½ tsp ground cinnamon
- pinch of salt

1. Preheat the oven to 400°F/200°C. Grease a 12-hole muffin tin or use paper cases.

2. Beat the eggs and sugar together until combined. Whisk in the bananas, buttermilk, bran, oil, vanilla essence, and cinnamon leaf oil.

3. Mix together the remaining dry ingredients, pour in the egg and sugar mixture, and stir.

4. Spoon into the muffin tin and bake for 15 minutes until firm to touch. Cool on a wire rack before eating.

Life affirming

Psychologically, cinnamon leaf is fortifying and reviving, indicated for nervous exhaustion and general debility. Cinnamon leaf is life affirming, helping to alleviate depression characterized by lethargy and lack of vitality. Cinnamon leaf restores zest for life, and inspires courage.

CLOVE BUD

Syzgium aromaticum

*Botanical Family:
Myrtaceae*

Clove was a traditional ingredient of ancient Egyptian fragrances, and in small amounts adds a harmonizing, mysterious, and oriental dimension to perfumes.

METHOD OF EXTRACTION:
Clove bud essential oil is water distilled from the flower buds.

REGIONS OF ORIGIN:
Indonesia, Madagascar, Philippines, Tanzania.

CHARACTERISTICS:
Clove bud is a pale yellow thin essential oil that easily drops from the bottle dropper.

FRAGRANCE DESCRIPTION:
Clove bud has fresh, fruity top notes and deep, sweet, warm, spicy, undertones.

SAFE USAGE: Do not use if you have sensitive or very sensitive skin. Use no more than 2 drops in the bath, and use no more than 1% dilution in massage oils.

PLANT DESCRIPTION

Clove is a long-lived evergreen tree, which grows to about 40 feet. It has a smooth gray trunk with glossy green leaves growing in pairs. When the rainy season begins, long, rosy pink buds appear that become fragrant red flowers with purple fruits. These are beaten down from the tree and dried to produce the familiar clove bud.

BLENDING PROFILE

In tiny amounts, clove bud blends well with most citrus and floral oils, and also with clary sage, bay, palmarosa, lemongrass, benzoin, and sandalwood.

TRADITIONAL USES

The clove tree is indigenous to the Molucca Islands and formed an important part of their spice trade. Clove has always had a high commercial value and continues to do so today. As well as clove bud essential oil, there are also clove leaf and clove stem essential oils. However, the latter two contain levels of chemicals unsafe for topical application so are not used in aromatherapy.

Over its long history, clove bud has been used as a tincture to treat scabies and athlete's foot, and to dress the newly cut umbilical cords of babies. A tea containing cloves relieves digestive upsets and also helps to get rid of intestinal parasites.

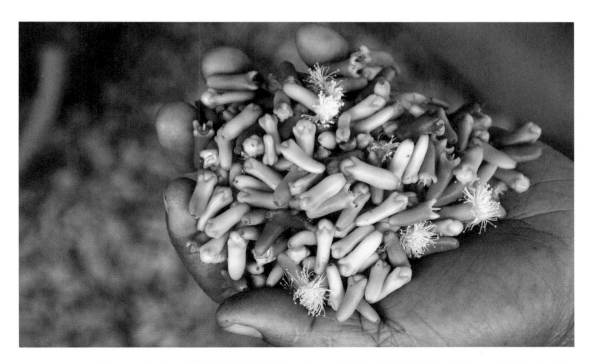

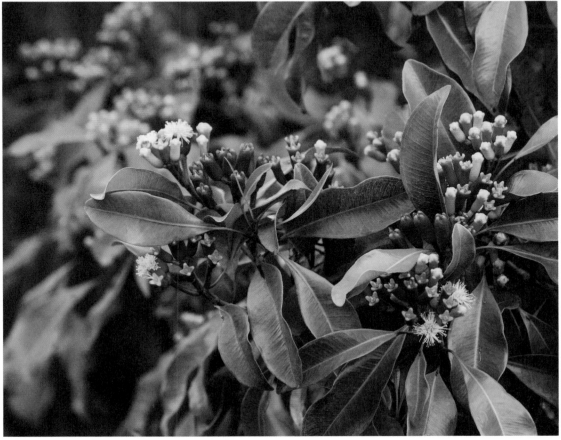

As well as the familiar culinary uses of clove, it is also used in the fragrance and pharmaceutical industries, including dental products. In Traditional Chinese Medicine clove is used for halitosis, hernia, diarrhea, and bronchitis.

THERAPEUTIC PROPERTIES

Analgesic, antibacterial, antiseptic, antispasmodic, carminative, stimulant, and stomachic. *(See glossary on page 158.)*

Tooth remedy

Clove bud has always been the first choice for emergency toothache. A couple of drops of clove bud on a cotton wool ball applied to an aching tooth has an anesthetic affect, relieving pain for a few hours. If the pain is caused by a lost filling, a piece of cotton wool soaked in clove and inserted into the cavity will have the same analgesic and anesthetic effect.

Antiseptic and pain-relieving

Its strong antiseptic properties make clove bud good at preventing colds and flu, and for these cases it is best diffused in a burner. Clove bud's antiseptic strength also makes it useful for a wide range of conditions, such as in a skin toner for treating acne and compresses over abscesses. Its analgesic property makes clove bud good in a cold compress over sprains and strains to reduce pain. Overall, clove bud is pain relieving, comforting, and revitalizing.

Restorative and stimulating

Small amounts of clove bud blended into massage oils can help relieve stiff, aching muscles, rheumatic joint pain, and neuralgia. If you feel "chilled to the bone," adding a couple of drops of clove to a bath-oil blend is warming and comforting. Clove bud works well on the digestive tract, helping relieve flatulence, stimulating digestion, and restoring appetite. Psychologically, clove bud is a mental, emotional, and subtle energy tonic, and is both restorative and stimulating.

Hot spiced cider

This is a warming and comforting drink that is perfect for cold, damp evenings. The addition of cloves and other spices helps fend off winter chills. If you don't drink alcohol or you want to serve the drink to children, use alcohol-free cider, or apple juice.

You will need:

- 2.5 ltr apple cider
- 2 cups fresh orange juice
- ½ cup fresh lemon juice
- 10 whole cloves
- 4 cinnamon sticks
- 1-in (2½-cm) piece ginger root, chopped
- pinch of ground nutmeg
- 4 drops organic clove bud essential oil

1. Put the cider, orange juice, and lemon juice in a large pan over a low heat, and stir to combine. Once the cider is steaming hot, add all the spices and clove bud essential oil.

2. Bring to the boil and simmer for 10 minutes. Remove the whole spices and taste; you can add sugar if you like. Serve hot.

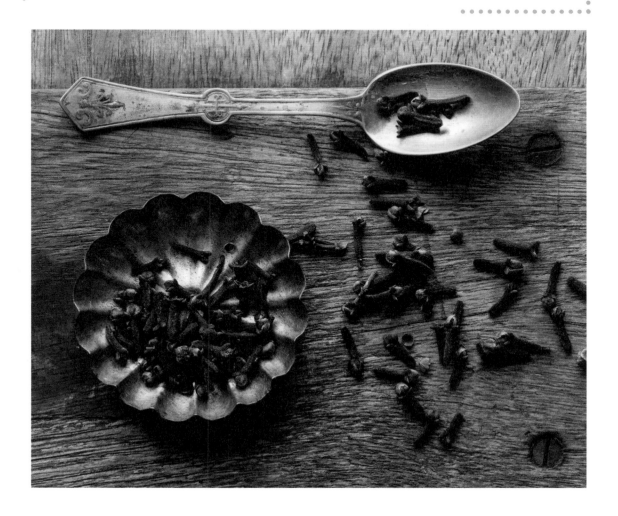

NUTMEG

Myristica fragrans

*Botanical Family:
Myristicaceae*

Nutmeg is good in massage blends for painful muscles and joints, as it is warming and analgesic.

METHOD OF EXTRACTION:
Nutmeg essential oil is steam or water distilled from dried nutmegs after worms have eaten away all the starch and fat.

REGIONS OF ORIGIN:
Grenada, Indonesia,
Sri Lanka, West Indies.

CHARACTERISTICS:
Nutmeg is a pale yellow or clear thin essential oil.

FRAGRANCE DESCRIPTION:
Nutmeg has light, pungent, spicy top notes and deep, sweet, warm, woody undertones.

SAFE USAGE: Avoid during pregnancy. Use in moderation, and not consistently over long periods of time.

PLANT DESCRIPTION

Nutmeg is an aromatic, evergreen rainforest tree.

BLENDING PROFILE

Nutmeg blends well with other spice oils, and also with clary sage, mandarin, sweet orange, geranium, lavender, rose, jasmine, rosemary, lemongrass, lime, and petitgrain.

TRADITIONAL USES

Nutmeg has a long history of use as a culinary spice and also as a remedy for digestive problems. Nutmeg is also used extensively in the food, fragrance, and pharmaceutical industries.

THERAPEUTIC PROPERTIES

Analgesic, antirheumatic, antiseptic, antispasmodic, aphrodisiac, digestive, emmenagogue, carminative, rubefacient, stimulant, and tonic. *(See glossary on page 158.)*

Euphoric and comforting
Blended with floral and citrus oils, its aphrodisiac properties make nutmeg useful in sensuous massage blends for lovers. Nutmeg can also help poor digestion, nausea, and diarrhea. Overall, nutmeg is euphoric, comforting, and elevating.

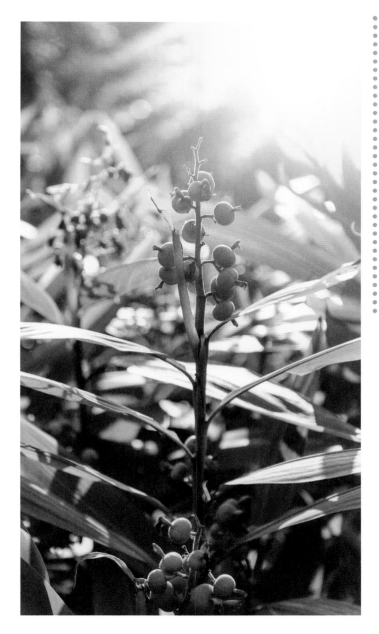

Nutmeg baked rice pudding

Rice pudding is nutritious and easy to digest. Freshly grated nutmeg adds an exotic, spicy flavor.

You will need:
- 3 tbsp butter
- ½ cup pudding rice
- ½ cup superfine sugar
- 1¾ pt (1 ltr) whole milk
- ⅔ cup half-and-half cream
- pinch of salt
- 1 tsp vanilla essence
- freshly grated nutmeg

1. Preheat the oven to 285°F/140°C. Melt the butter in a pan over a medium heat, add the rice and stir well.

2. After 5 minutes add the sugar and keep stirring till the sugar has dissolved and the rice has become sticky and is beginning to swell.

3. Add the milk, turn up the heat, stirring continuously until the mixture begins to boil.

4. Turn down, add the cream, salt and vanilla essence, and stir well.

5. Pour into a large buttered casserole dish, grate lots of fresh nutmeg over the top and bake for 1 hour.

Nerve tonic

Psychologically, nutmeg is an uplifting nerve tonic, relieving chronic fatigue, debility, anxiety, and depression, and comforting those who feel at the end of their tether. Nutmeg is useful in meditations for those who are both sleepy tired and tired of life.

PETITGRAIN

Citrus aurantium

Botanical Family:
Rutaceae

Petitgrain is a traditional ingredient of eau de Cologne, and is included in many other perfumes. It is also used to scent soaps.

METHOD OF EXTRACTION:
Petitgrain is steam distilled from the leaves; sometimes small twigs are also included, although this produces an inferior oil.

REGIONS OF ORIGIN:
Algeria, France, Haiti, Italy, Paraguay.

CHARACTERISTICS:
Petitgrain is a pale yellow thin oil that easily drops from the bottle dropper. It shares many of the therapeutic qualities of neroli and has a similar, though less fine, scent.

FRAGRANCE DESCRIPTION:
Petitgrain has fresh, sweet, floral, citrussy top notes with light, woody, herbaceous undertones.

SAFE USAGE: Petitgrain is a safe, easy-to-use essential oil.

PLANT DESCRIPTION

Petitgrain—also known as petitgrain bigarade—is produced from the bitter orange tree, which is also called the Seville orange. It is an evergreen tree, native to Southeast Asia, but is now mainly cultivated in the Mediterranean countries. It has dark green leaves and fragrant white flowers.

BLENDING PROFILE

Petitgrain blends well with most floral and citrus oils, as well as rosemary, thyme, clary sage, black pepper, ginger, benzoin, patchouli, palmarosa, and cardamom.

TRADITIONAL USES

The word petitgrain comes from the French, meaning "little seed." Petitgrain from France is called petitgrain bigarade and is considered much finer than the petitgrain from Paraguay, which has a stronger but much less refined odor.

THERAPEUTIC PROPERTIES

Antibacterial, antiseptic, anti-inflammatory, anti-infectious, antispasmodic, deodorant, digestive, nervine, stomachic, and sedative. *(See glossary on page 158.)*

Balancing and refreshing

The refreshing properties of petitgrain are often used in skin and haircare products, particularly for infected or

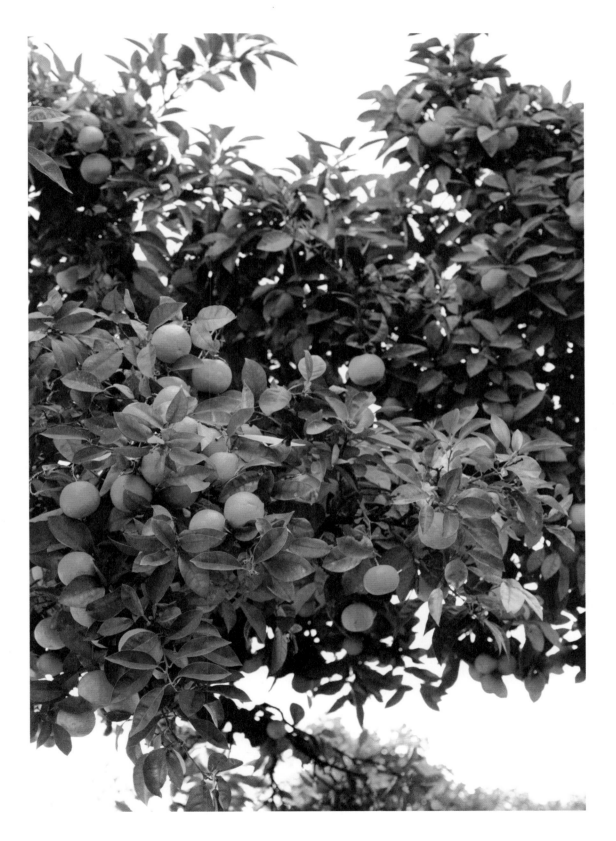

severe acne, and to help balance oily skin and greasy hair. Petitgrain helps clear blemishes and reduce overactive sebum production, and is particularly effective in facial treatments, when blended with geranium. Overall, petitgrain has a relaxing, balancing, refreshing quality.

Petitgrain is recommended for nervous tension and anxiety, and is even more effective for these emotional issues when blended with neroli. It is also helpful against rheumatic pain caused or aggravated by nervous tension. Petitgrain is similar to but less effective than neroli in many therapeutic remedies, but is considerably cheaper.

Promotes sleep

When added to your evening bath—perhaps blended with Roman chamomile, sweet marjoram, or lavender—petitgrain helps prevent insomnia, especially if you are sad or lonely. It can be used in massage blends, both for local and full body massage, to treat dyspepsia and help digestion. In a chest rub blended with niaouli, pine needles, and frankincense, petitgrain is also good for respiratory infections.

Calming and meditative

Psychologically, petitgrain is revitalizing, balancing, and nourishing, and clears away troubled emotions. Petitgrain is a sedative and helps ease a troubled mind. It is good in a meditation blend to help you get in touch with the rational and intellectual mind. Petitgrain's soft, delicate, gentle aroma is useful in convalescence, especially when a stronger fragrance would be overwhelming.

Holistic petitgrain blends

This holistic recipe for petitgrain is called "reuniting the whole," meaning it uses other essential oils from the same orange tree. So, it also includes either sweet orange or bitter orange from the fruit and neroli, also known as orange flower blossom, from the flowers. The combination of these three essential oils from the same plant are more than the sum of their parts. This is called synergy in aromatherapy; when you create blends of related essential oils, or those that have a particular affinity together, and the effect is more than you would logically expect from the combination of the actual ingredients. This concept of synergy is part of the magical, spiritual side of aromatherapy.

Available from natural health stores, base products are perfume and color free and are used to make your own blends. Mix the essential oils thoroughly into the base product.

You will need:

- 3 drops petitgrain essential oil
- 3 drops sweet or bitter orange essential oil
- 2 drops neroli essential oil

To make body lotion: Mix this combination of essential oil drops into 4 tsp base lotion in a 1 fl oz (25 ml) dark glass jar.

To make hand cream: Mix this combination of essential oil drops into 4 tsp base cream in a 1 fl oz (25 ml) dark glass jar. Then stir in 1 tsp melted shea butter.

To make bath oil (for two baths): Mix this combination of essential oil drops into 2 tsp dispersant base bath oil in a ½ fl oz (10 ml) glass bottle.

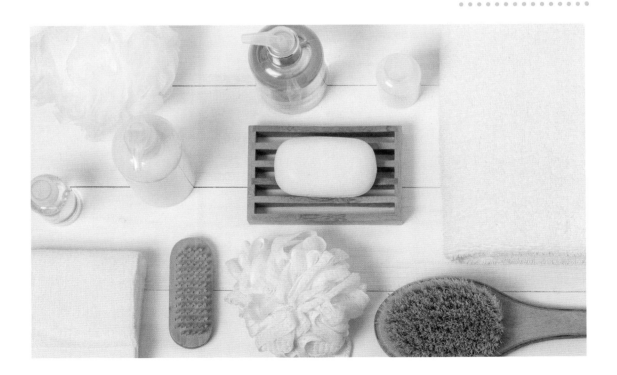

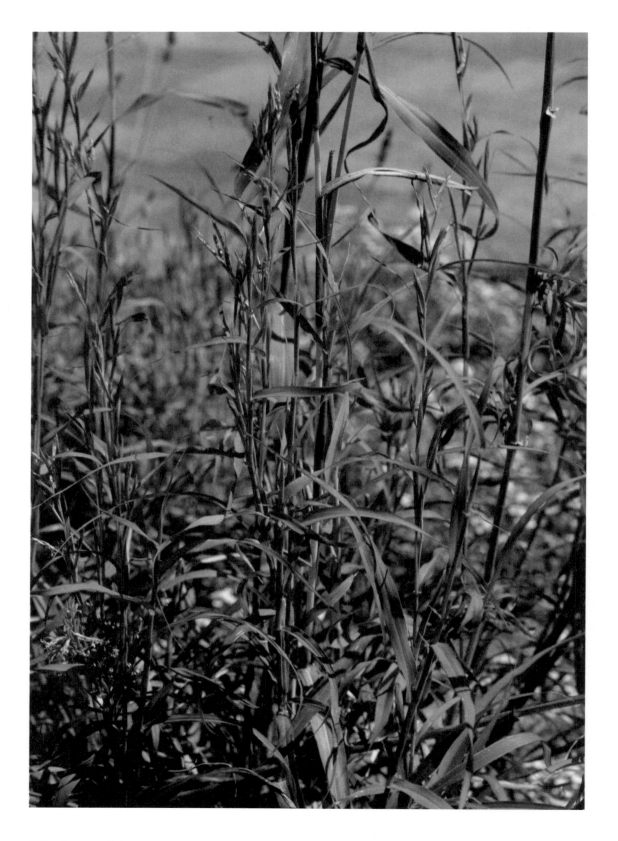

PALMAROSA

Cymbopogon martini

Botanical Family:
Poaceae (Gramineae)

Palmarosa is extensively used in modern perfumery and cosmetics, particularly in soaps, for its delicious fragrance and skin-enhancing properties.

METHOD OF EXTRACTION:
Palmarosa is steam distilled from the fresh or dried grass of mostly wild plants. The older leaves contain a higher oil content than young leaves.

REGIONS OF ORIGIN:
Africa, Brazil, Comoros Islands, India, Java, Pakistan, Seychelles, Southeast Asia.

CHARACTERISTICS:
Palmarosa is a pale yellow or olive thin oil that easily drops from the bottle dropper.

FRAGRANCE DESCRIPTION:
Palmerosa has sweet, light, floral top notes with subtle lemon, grassy, and rose geranium undertones. It has a complex fragrance that varies according to where it is grown.

SAFE USAGE: Palmarosa is a safe essential oil with no contraindications.

PLANT DESCRIPTION

Palmarosa is closely related to lemongrass and citronella, and all three essential oils are used in aromatherapy. Despite their striking similarity, each of these plants produces quite different essential oils with unique therapeutic properties. Palmarosa is a perennial and very aromatic herbaceous grass with stiff, upright yellow-green stems; its long, narrow leaves are a paler green than the stems. It can reach to over 8 feet in height when allowed to grow freely. In India palmarosa is called *russa*, *rohisha*, or *rosha* grass.

BLENDING PROFILE

Palmarosa blends well with citrus oils, and also with sweet basil, cedarwood atlas, sweet fennel, frankincense, rose, geranium, lavender, lemongrass, neroli, pine needles, and ylang ylang.

TRADITIONAL USES

Palmarosa has been used medicinally and as an insect repellent for thousands of years. In India the fresh leaves were crushed and used in bath water to soothe a tired mind and aching body. Palmarosa was also used in poultices to relieve pain from lumbagao, sciatica, rheumatism, and neuralgia. Palmarosa essential oil is still used today in massage oils for these purposes. In Indian Ayurvedic medicine, both grass and roots are made into a decoction and taken internally to treat bronchitis, coughs, and other respiratory disorders, and also to help relieve colitis, dyspepsia, fevers, and jaundice. For many years palmarosa was also used to flavor tobacco.

THERAPEUTIC PROPERTIES

Antiseptic, antifungal, antiviral, bactericide, cicatrisant, cytophylactic, digestive, febrifuge, and tonic. *(See glossary on page 158.)*

Useful during convalescence

Palmarosa has a powerful antimicrobial action, reputed to be even stronger than tea tree, and its antifungal properties help treat athlete's foot and other fungal infections. A good digestive stimulant, palmarosa is recommended in local massage and baths for sluggish digestion and loss of appetite. It is also traditionally used to combat digestive infections, and is useful during convalescence.

Used in massage blends, palmarosa eases the pain associated with arthritis, rheumatism, and general muscular aches, as well as cramps and gastric conditions. Owing to its calming yet uplifting properties, palmarosa is valuable when treating emotional conditions such as anxiety, nervous exhaustion, and stress. Palmarosa is especially effective when blended with lavender, vetivert, and rose.

Balancing and hydrating

Palmarosa is much used in all skincare preparations for its lovely fragrance, and its sebum balancing and hydrating properties. It also helps regenerate skin cells, thereby maintaining a fresh and radiant complexion. Palmarosa is suited to all skin types, but is especially good for dry, mature, and damaged skin. This makes it a useful addition to face creams, body lotions, body butters, and hand creams, as well as face washes and scrubs. It is also effective at combating acne and soothing dermatitis, eczema, and psoriasis. Overall, palmarosa is balancing, refreshing, and calming.

Psychologically, palmarosa is uplifting and comforting and is useful for all kinds of stress, tension, anxiety, and restlessness, especially when these emotions have left you feeling vulnerable, lonely, and insecure.

Moisturizing face wash

This foaming cleanser is fragranced with palmarosa and lavender; both of which were traditionally used for washing. It leaves your skin clean, hydrated, and radiant.

You will need:

- 1 cup foaming bath butter
- 1 tbsp sweet almond oil
- 3 drops palmarosa essential oil
- 3 drops lavender essential oil
- ½–1 tsp Rhassoul Lava clay (or green or pink clay)

1. Place the foaming bath butter in a bowl and beat with an electric hand mixer until doubled in size.

2. Add the palmarosa and lavender oils to the almond oil, tip into the bowl and beat again until fully incorporated.

3. Fold in the clay with a spoon until the mixture looks even. Spoon into a jar and label.

4. To use the wash, work a little into your moistened skin—it will foam like soap—and then rinse off with water. Your skin will be deeply cleansed and feel beautifully hydrated.

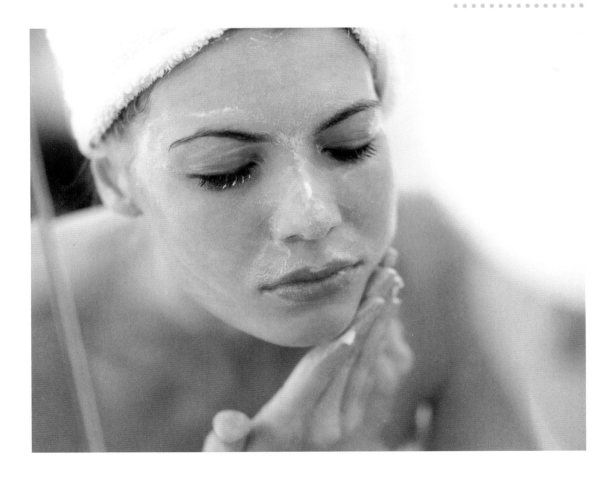

PATCHOULI

Pogostemom cablin

Botanical Family:
Lamiaceae (Labiatae)

Psychologically, patchouli is soothing, stabilizing, and slightly hypnotic. It is excellent for reducing stress and alleviating anxiety and depression.

METHOD OF EXTRACTION:
Patchouli essential oil is steam distilled from the dried, fermented leaves.

REGIONS OF ORIGIN:
China, India, Indonesia, Malaysia, Mauritius, Philippines, west Africa, West Indies, Vietnam.

CHARACTERISTICS:
Patchouli is a dark orange or amber brown, slightly viscous oil that easily drops from the bottle dropper.

FRAGRANCE DESCRIPTION:
Patchouli has warm, rich, sweet, spicy, woody top notes and earthy, herbaceous, musky, balsamic undertones. The fragrance of this essential oil is extremely tenacious and improves with age.

SAFE USAGE: Patchouli is a safe essential oil.

PLANT DESCRIPTION

Patchouli is an aromatic, perennial shrub reaching over 3 feet at maturity. It has large, furry green leaves, and white-pink flowers with purple edges.

BLENDING PROFILE

Patchouli blends well with lavender, vetivert, sandalwood, cedarwood atlas, rose, neroli, jasmine, ylang ylang, lemon, bergamot, sweet orange, lime, mandarin, grapefruit, geranium, myrrh, frankincense, and clary sage.

TRADITIONAL USES

Patchouli is widely used throughout Asia in incense, to repel insects, as a body and garment fragrance, and ceremonially in temples. In India patchouli was used to perfume textiles; in Arabia to perfume carpets; and in ancient China to produce a fragrant ink. In the 19th century, when cloth and clothes began to be imported to Europe in large quantities, coarsely ground patchouli was scattered between the layers. Although the purpose was to repel insects, the fragrance became popular and this culminated in its use by hippies in the 1960s.

In traditional Chinese medicine patchouli is sometimes used to treat colds, headaches, nausea, vomiting, and abdominal pain. Elsewhere, it is used extensively in both the perfume and cosmetics industries.

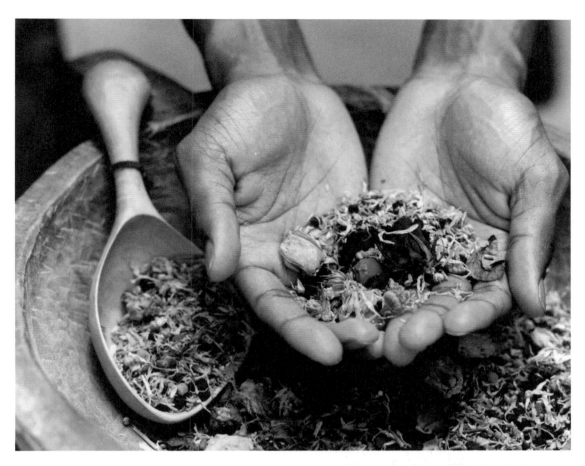

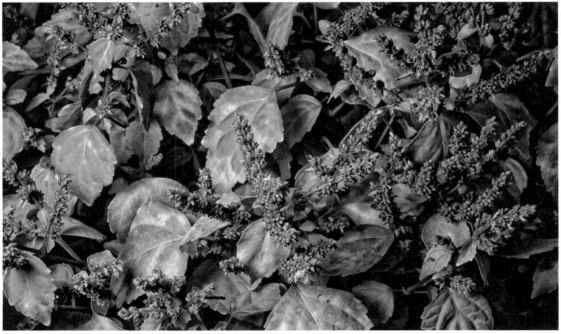

THERAPEUTIC PROPERTIES

Antidepressant, anti–inflammatory, antimicrobial, antiphlogistic, antitoxic, aphrodisiac, antiseptic, astringent, cicatrisant, cytophylactic, deodorant, diuretic, febrifuge, fungicide, insecticide, and sedative. *(See glossary on page 158.)*

Aphrodisiac qualities

Patchouli is a powerful aphrodisiac, and adds a sensuous, erotic, oriental note to perfumes. However, not everyone likes its distinctive scent; for those who don't, it is definitely not an aphrodisiac! Overall, patchouli is relaxing, uplifting, and sensual.

Hydrating and cooling

Excellent in skincare products, patchouli is regenerating, hydrating, and cooling: It heals inflammation, dermatitis, sores, eczema, and other skin conditions. Patchouli is particularly suited to mature and oily skins and helps regenerate healthy new skin cells. It is often included in anti-aging face serums to combat wrinkles. When blended into wheatgerm oil, it helps reduce the visibility of scar tissue. Patchouli also makes a good addition to base shampoo and conditioner, helping alleviate dandruff and an itchy scalp.

Patchouli is good in massage blends, and helps those who are overly intellectual, bringing them in touch with their earthy, sensual nature. It grounds those who get lost in daydreams, and is good in meditation for calming too many thoughts and bringing stillness to the mind.

Potpourri

This recipe uses patchouli in the traditional way to fragrance rooms and protect against insects. The tenacity means the potpourri will last a long time and the all-natural ingredients avoids the chemicals of commercial air fresheners, which have been identified as potential allergens.

If you find the scent of patchouli overwhelming, use a blend including other lighter essential oils. For example, 4 drops patchouli essential oil, 2 drops lavender essential oil, 2 drops mandarin essential oil, and 2 drops geranium essential oil.

You will need:

- small handful each dried rose buds or petals, lavender buds, marigold flowers, bay leaves, rosemary sprigs, or eucalyptus leaves, or a mixture of other fragrant dried herbs and flowers
- 8–10 drops patchouli essential oil

1. Create your mix of dried herbs and flowers and place in a small ornamental bowl.

2. Drip on the patchouli, and other oils if using a blend, and mix into the dried herbs with a spoon.

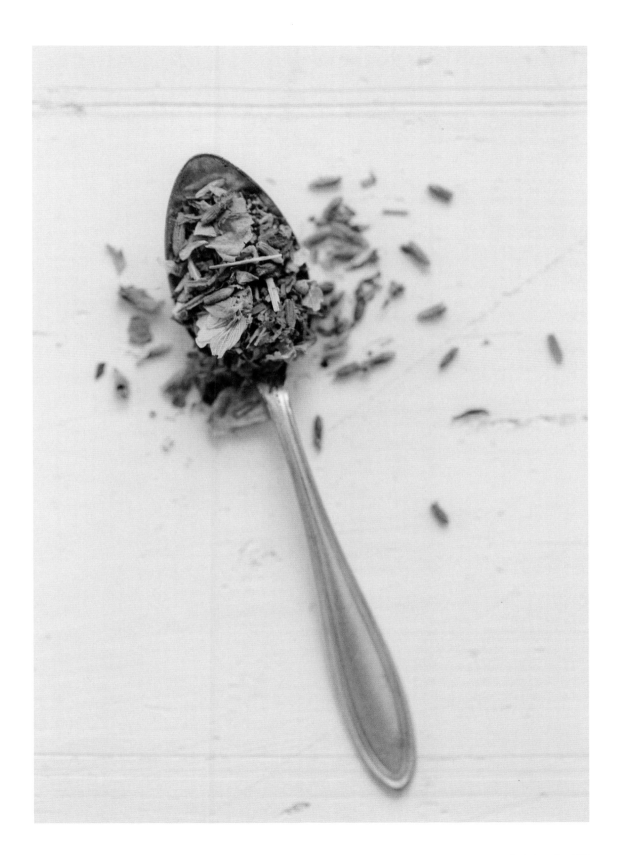

LEMONGRASS

Cymbopogon citratus, Cymbopogon flexuosus

Botanical Family:
Poaceae (Gramineae)

Lemongrass is an excellent deodorant, which makes it a good choice to use in a burner to clear and freshen the air.

METHOD OF EXTRACTION:
The essential oil is steam distilled from finely chopped fresh, or partly dried, grass.

REGIONS OF ORIGIN:
Africa, Argentina, Brazil, Burma, Comoros Islands, Guatemala, Honduras, India, Madagascar, Malaysia, Sri Lanka, Thailand, Vietnam.

CHARACTERISTICS:
Lemongrass is a yellow or amber, slightly viscous oil that easily drops from the bottle dropper.

FRAGRANCE DESCRIPTION:
Lemongrass has pungent, fresh, lemon sherbet, hay-like top notes with earthy, green grassy, lemon undertones.

SAFE USAGE: Do not use on sensitive skin. Use maximum 3 drops in the bath; maximum 2% dilution in massage oils.

PLANT DESCRIPTION

There are two types of lemongrass: *Cymbopogon citratus* is known as West Indian or Guatemala lemongrass, and *Cymbopogon flexuosus* is known as East Indian lemongrass. The plant is a tall, aromatic, perennial, fast-growing grass, which rarely flowers. The two varieties are distinct species, but share similar properties.

BLENDING PROFILE

Lemongrass blends well with most citrus and floral oils, and also with sweet marjoram, black pepper, rosemary, clary sage, cardamom, and ginger.

TRADITIONAL USES

Lemongrass has always been used to flavor food, and the leaves were crushed in water and used on the hair and skin. In Indian folk medicine lemongrass was used against infectious disease and to cool fever. The essential oil is used to produce citral, a natural component of lemongrass, for use in the perfume, flavor, and pharmaceutical industries. West Indian lemongrass is used in Traditional Chinese Medicine.

THERAPEUTIC PROPERTIES

Analgesic, antibacterial, antidepressant, antimicrobial, antiseptic, astringent, bactericide, carminative, deodorant, febrifuge, fungicidal, insecticidal, nervine, sedative, toning, and tonic. *(See glossary on page 158.)*

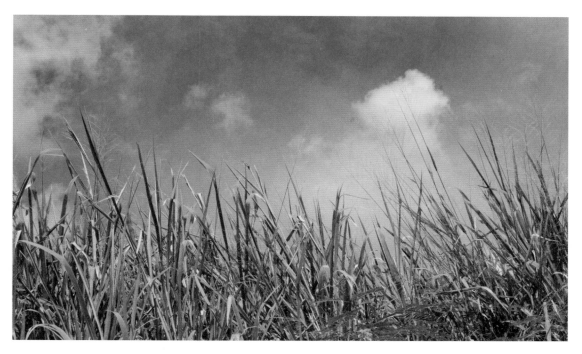

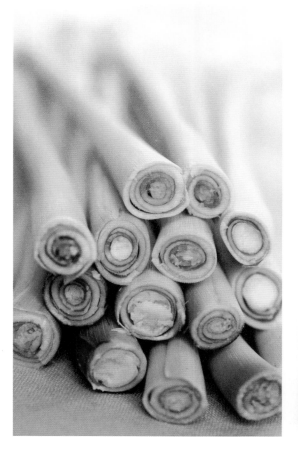

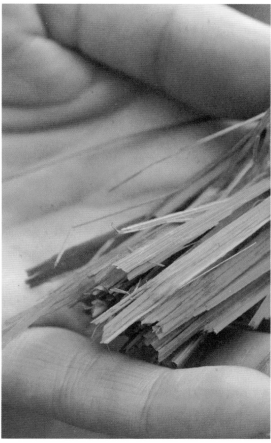

Tones connective tissue

Lemongrass is sometimes called the connective-tissue essential oil, as it tightens and tones the skin and connective tissue. This makes it useful in massage and compresses after sports injuries, over-training or overdoing it in the gym, general strains, and sprains, and also after dieting when the connective tissues and skin may have lost tone and become slack. Overall, lemongrass is cooling, refreshing, and stimulating.

Powerful antiseptic

Lemongrass is good in skincare, as its toning action helps reduce open pores and rebalance overactive sebaceous glands. This makes it useful for treating oily skin and helping clear up and reduce spots and acne. Lemongrass is a powerful antiseptic and this, along with its antiviral and antifungal properties, makes it useful for treating athlete's foot and other fungal and bacterial infections. Added to a shampoo or conditioner base, lemongrass stimulates the hair follicles thereby promoting hair growth, and also stimulating hair regrowth.

Soothes headaches

Lemongrass is soothing for headaches, but should be properly diluted before applying to the temples, and is particularly good blended with lavender. It is also an effective digestive stimulant and recommended for colitis, indigestion, and gastroenteritis.

Psychologically, lemongrass is uplifting and energizing. It is especially good to get you going in the morning: A few drops sprinkled in the shower will vaporize in the hot water and steam, surrounding you with fragrant energy. Lemongrass is helpful for concentration and clear thinking, so it is useful in a burner when you are studying or meditating.

Lemongrass ginger tea

Lemongrass is a beneficial tonic for the digestive system when drunk as an infusion, and this tea also helps eliminate toxins. This simple-to-make tisane is useful if you are dieting, detoxifying, or simply want to give your system a morning cleanse.

You will need:

- 1 lemongrass bulb
- 1-in (2½-cm) piece ginger root
- honey to sweeten, if desired
- 1 cup boiling water

1. Wash, chop, and bruise the lemongrass and ginger to release the essential oils and other nutrients.

2. Place in a pan and add the boiling water.

3. Bring back to the boil, turn the heat down, cover, and simmer for 10 minutes.

4. Strain into a mug, taste, and add a little honey to sweeten, if desired.

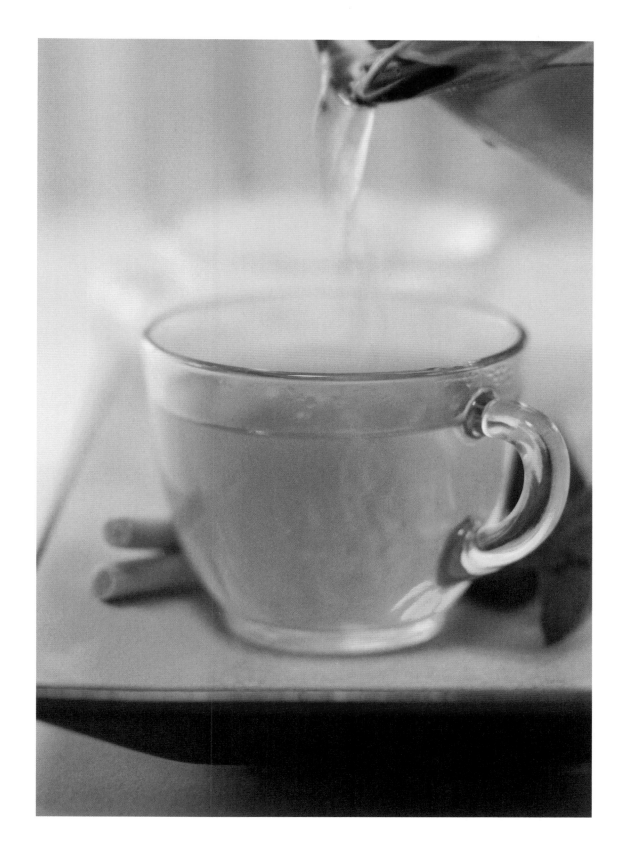

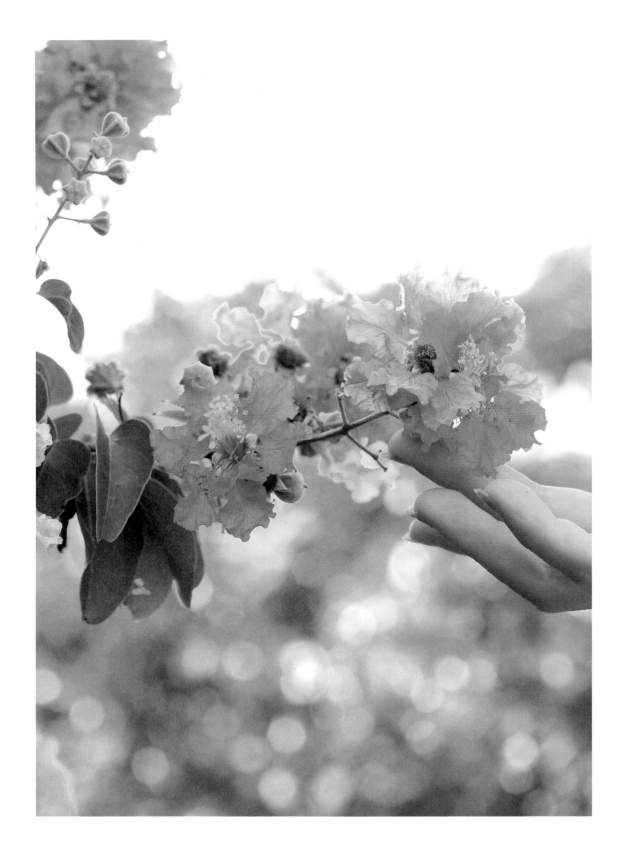

MYRTLE

Myrtus communis

Botanical Family:
Myrtaceae

Myrtle is one of the best essential oils for children's ailments, as it is mildly sedative and has a gentle action, as well as a soft, pleasing fragrance.

METHOD OF EXTRACTION:
Myrtle essential oil is steam distilled from the leaves and twigs; sometimes the flowers are also included.

REGIONS OF ORIGIN:
Corsica, France, Italy, Morocco, Spain, Tunisia.

CHARACTERISTICS:
Myrtle is a pale yellow, orange or greenish thin essential oil that easily drops from the bottle dropper.

FRAGRANCE DESCRIPTION:
Myrtle has warm, fresh, spicy, camphoraceous top notes and floral, herbaceous, woody undertones. Its fragrance is similar to eucalyptus, but softer.

SAFE USAGE: Myrtle is a safe essential oil, and often used in the treatment of children.

PLANT DESCRIPTION

Myrtle is an evergreen shrub or small tree with red-brown bark, small, pointed, fragrant leaves, and intensely fragrant white or pink flowers, followed by small purple-black berries.

BLENDING PROFILE

Myrtle blends well with spice oils, also lavender, neroli, lime, bergamot, lemon, hyssop, bay, rosemary, clary sage, pine needles, and cypress.

TRADITIONAL USES

Myrtle has a long tradition of use in herbal medicine. The leaves were steeped in wine and used to treat afflictions, such as lung and bronchial infections and urinary tract infections. Both leaves and berries were used to treat diarrhea, dysentery, and congested catarrhal chest conditions and tuberculosis; the action of the leaves and berries was considered drying and binding.

Myrtle flowers and leaves were also included in "angels' water," a 16th-century skincare preparation. In Italy myrtle was used in children's cough syrups.

THERAPEUTIC PROPERTIES

Anticatarrhal, antiseptic, astringent, bactericide, balsamic, expectorant, and mildly sedative. *(See glossary on page 158.)*

Alleviates coughs

Myrtle is especially recommended for respiratory ailments, and is good in back and chest massage, baths, and steam inhalations. At night in a child's bedroom, a burner of myrtle—placed out of reach—is settling, and alleviates irritable coughing. Because it has such a gentle action, myrtle is often preferred over other similar essential oils that have a stronger action, such as tea tree and eucalyptus, but it strengthens the immune system just as effectively. This is particularly important when treating children, weakened invalids, or elderly people for coughs, bronchitis, and other respiratory conditions.

Brightens skin

Its astringent property makes myrtle useful in skincare for oily skin, general skin irritations, spots, acne, and open pores, and it has a brightening effect on tired, lackluster skin. Myrtle is good blended with cypress into an ointment base for hemorrhoids. It can be used in a douche or hot compress over the kidneys to help treat urinary tract infections. Overall, myrtle is soothing, calming, and cheering.

Clarifying and protective

Psychologically, myrtle is clarifying, purifying, and protective. It has been recommended for addictive, self-destructive, compulsive, and obsessive behavior, especially if this manifests in drug use. Massage from an aromatherapist as part of a professional team is recommended for all serious cases. However, for minor and temporary instances, myrtle in massage, bath, and perfume blends can be supportive, particularly when blended with clary sage, bergamot, and neroli.

Myrtle is considered to be a quite spiritual essential oil and is reputed to carry the spirit of truth and forgiveness. Myrtle acts like a doorway to universal divine energies, so is useful in meditation blends.

Skin toner

This refreshing, astringent skin toner is a modern version of the traditional "angels' water" from the 16th century, but is much simpler to make. It is designed to tone and tighten the pores, prevent acne and spots developing, or prevent existing spots getting worse or infected, and to help improve oily skin. The fragrance of the skin toner will appeal to both women and men as it is not sweet and flowery, but neither is it too obviously masculine smelling.

You will need:

- 1 x 3½ fl oz (100 ml) dark glass bottle
- 1 tsp perfumer's alcohol (see page 40)
- 3½ fl oz (100 ml) orange flower water
- 3½ fl oz (100 ml) witch hazel
- 10 drops myrtle essential oil
- 2 drops geranium essential oil
- 3 drops bergamot essential oil
- 2 drops juniper berry essential oil
- 1 drop neroli essential oil
- 2 drops lavender essential oil

1. Measure the perfumer's alcohol and pour into the bottle.

2. Carefully drop in the required number of drops of each essential oil into the bottle and swish around to disperse.

3. Top up with the orange flower water and the witch hazel and swish around again to thoroughly mix all the ingredients together.

4. Label the bottle with the ingredients, amounts used, and date.

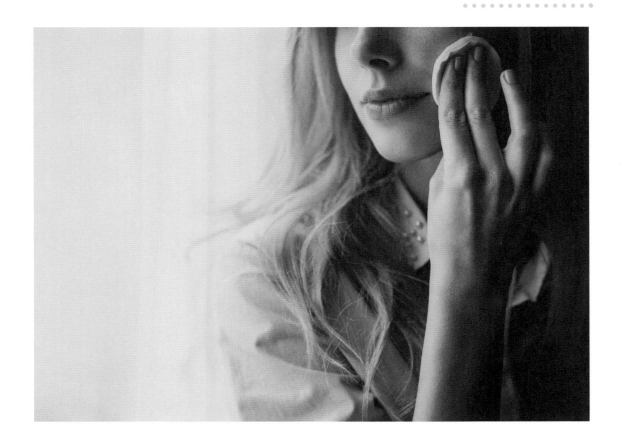

FRANKINCENSE

Boswellia carterii, Boswellia frereana, Boswellia serrata

Botanical Family:
Burseraceae

All the frankincense varieties slow and deepen breathing, helping to allay fear, anxiety, nervous tension, and stress.

METHOD OF EXTRACTION:
Frankincense is an oleo-gum-resin. Incisions into the bark of the Burseraceae tree produce a milky white resin that hardens into brown resin "tears," from which the essential oil is steam distilled.

REGIONS OF ORIGIN:
Ethiopia, Oman, Saudi Arabia, Somalia, Yemen.

CHARACTERISTICS:
Frankincense is a pale yellow, thin essential oil that easily drops from the bottle dropper.

FRAGRANCE DESCRIPTION:
Frankincense generally has fresh, citrus, turpentine top notes and sweet, warm, balsamic, camphoraceous, wood-smoke undertones.

SAFE USAGE: Frankincense is a safe essential oil.

PLANT DESCRIPTION

There are several species of *Boswellia* used in aromatherapy, the most familiar being *carterii* which, along with *sacra* and *frereana*, usually comes from Somalia. *Papyifera* comes from western Ethiopia and *serrata* from western India. *Boswellia* are small, shrubby trees with white flowers.

BLENDING PROFILE

Frankincense blends well with most floral, wood, spice, and citrus oils, and also myrrh, patchouli, clary sage, rosemary, sweet basil, and vetivert.

TRADITIONAL USES

The name frankincense comes from Old French "*franc*" meaning free, pure or abundant, and Latin "*incensum*" meaning to smoke. Frankincense was historically important, playing a major role in ancient Egyptian, Persian, Hebrew, Greek, and Roman civilizations. It was used in incense and religious ceremonies and was an important cosmetic ingredient.

THERAPEUTIC PROPERTIES

Anti-inflammatory, antiseptic, astringent, carminative, cicatrisant, cytophylactic, diuretic, digestive, diuretic, emmenagogue, expectorant, sedative, uterine, tonic, and vulnerary. *(See glossary on page 158.)*

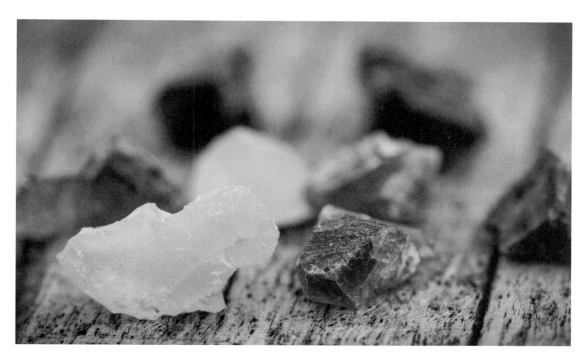

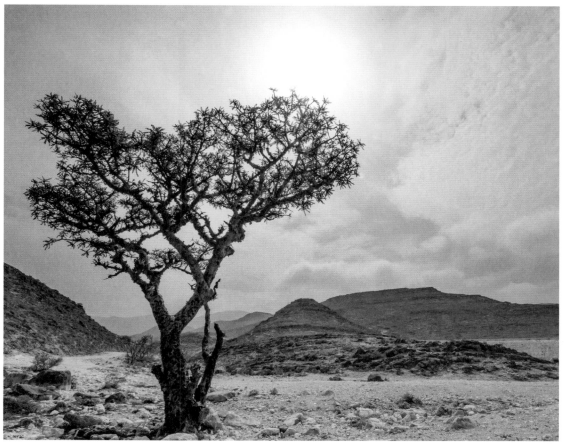

Benefits of frankincense varieties

Boswellia carterii is the most familiar frankincense essential oil. It has many therapeutic properties, such as supporting the immune system, and offers fantastic skincare properties, including reducing wrinkles. It also reduces the appearance of scars owing to its ability to repair skin cells. Its effect on the respiratory system is intriguing as frankincense slows and deepens the breathing; this explains why it is used to make incense. It has a deep, rich, heady aroma that quietens the mind and brings tranquility.

Boswellia frereana is grown at a high altitude in the mountains of Somalia. It is the best frankincense to relieve inflammation and pain caused by arthritis and to help with allergies.

Boswellia serrata is the oldest documented frankincense, and is probably the frankincense referred to in the Bible. This makes it excellent for meditation, and as a traditional anointing oil. Frankincense *serrata* has potent antiseptic, decongestant, and anti-inflammatory properties and is a good deodorant and air purifier. Its aroma is sweet and delicate, with clean, citrus, pine top notes.

Relieves anxiety

Frankincense is used to treat respiratory conditions, especially bronchitis, colds, sore throats, coughs, and catarrhal congestion. With asthma frankincense relieves the anxiety, deepens the breathing, and relieves the physical symptoms. Valuable in massage and bath oils, frankincense is also good in inhalations, burners, and perfumes. Frankincense is good in full body massage blends, bringing about a deep calm and relaxation. Overall, frankincense is calming, revitalizing, and uplifting.

Psychologically, frankincense inspires mystical, divine states, and stills the mind. It was traditionally used to drive away bad spirits, and it helps break links with the past.

Anti-aging eye cream

This eye cream helps dispel fine lines around the eyes.

You will need:

- a small dark glass jar
- 1 fl oz (25 ml) base cream
- 1 tsp aloe vera gel
- 4 drops rosehip seed oil
- 2 ml rose water
- 4 drops *Boswellia carterii* essential oil

1. Spoon the base cream into the jar, add the aloe vera gel and rose water. Stir with a chopstick or glass stirring rod until combined.

2. Add the drops of rosehip seed oil and frankincense and stir in well.

3. Label the jar with the ingredients, amounts used, and date.

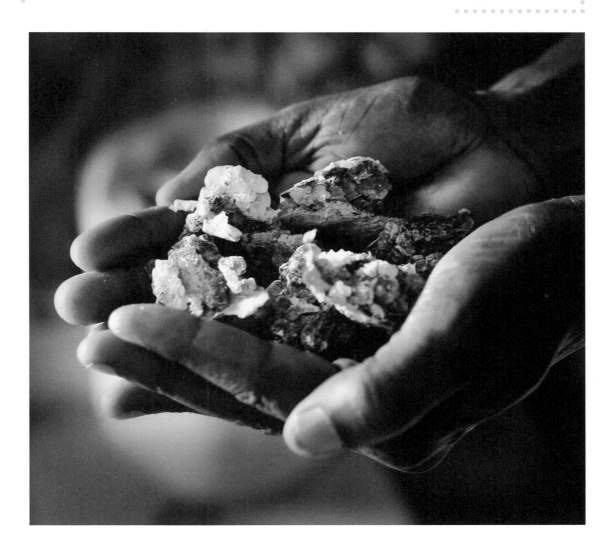

MYRRH

Commiphora myrrha

Botanical Family:
Burseraceae

Myrrh has been used in aromatherapy for over 4,000 years. The name comes from the Arabic *mur,* meaning bitter.

METHOD OF EXTRACTION:
Incisions into the bark produce a yellow resin that hardens into red brown "tears" from which the essential oil is steam distilled.

REGIONS OF ORIGIN:
Ethiopia, Somalia, Yemen.

CHARACTERISTICS:
Myrrh is a dark brown, amber, or yellow viscous essential oil that thickens with age. You may have to warm the bottle in hot water before the oil will drop out.

FRAGRANCE DESCRIPTION:
Myrhh has bitter, spicy, balsamic top notes and resinous, medicinal, sweet, wood smoke undertones.

SAFE USAGE: Avoid during pregnancy, otherwise safe.

PLANT DESCRIPTION

Myrrh is a shrubby bush growing up to 30 feet, with gnarled branches, aromatic leaves, and white flowers.

BLENDING PROFILE

Myrrh blends well with other resin oils, also patchouli, rose, sandalwood, mandarin, geranium, lavender, juniper berry, cypress, and pine needles.

TRADITIONAL USES

The ancient Egyptians used myrrh in religious ceremonies, incense, embalming, the perfume *kyphi*, and for face care. Ancient Greek soldiers carried it into battle for psychic protection and first aid. Traditional Chinese Medicine uses myrrh to stem bleeding, to relieve hemorrhoids, to bring on menstruation, relieve pain, and heal wounds. Myrrh is used in toothpastes, and mouth and throat gargles.

THERAPEUTIC PROPERTIES

Anti-catarrhal, anti-inflammatory, antimicrobial, antiseptic, astringent, balsamic, carminative, cicatrisant, digestive, emmenagogue, expectorant, fungicidal, pulmonary stimulant, stomachic, sedative, tonic, uterine, and vulnerary. *(See glossary on page 158.)*

Myrrh is first choice to treat athlete's foot, chronic wounds, ulcers, and gum infections, and it is frequently used as a tincture diluted in 70–80% alcohol. Mixed into a base ointment, myrrh treats hemorrhoids and minor bedsores. Overall, myrrh is healing, soothing, and gently restorative.

Skin healing

Blended into creams and serums, myrrh treats cracked, inflamed, and chapped skin and eczema. Reputed to reduce wrinkles, it revitalizes mature complexions, especially when blended with rose. Myrrh also treats coughs, bronchial conditions, and colds; it has a drying effect on excess mucous.

Psychologically, myrrh soothes stress and anxiety, inspiring peace and tranquility. It is excellent for meditation. Myrrh is associated with the base chakra, and helps people who are stuck to move on in life.

Healing foot gel

Myrrh's wound-healing ability and antifungal property make this a great gel for healing athlete's foot.

You will need:

- a small glass jar
- 1 tsp aloe vera gel
- 3 drops myrrh essential oil

1. Spoon the aloe vera gel into the jar and add the drops of myrrh. Mix together thoroughly.

2. Use up to four times a day until the infection has gone.

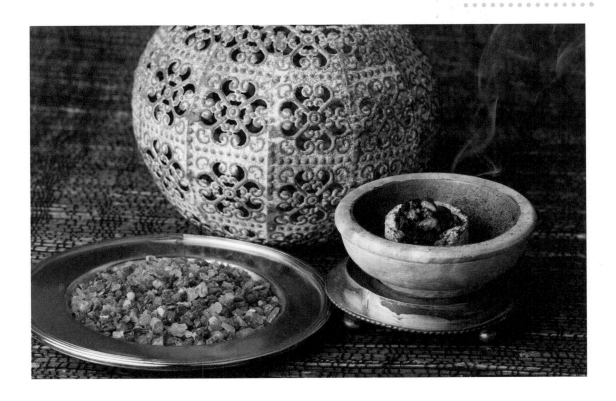

VETIVERT

Vetiveria zizanoides

Botanical Family:
Poaceae (Gramineae)

Vetivert is known as the oil of tranquility. Vetivert roots are traditionally woven into screens and mats to scent houses and repel moths.

METHOD OF EXTRACTION:
The essential oil is steam distilled from the washed, chopped roots, which are first dried to increase the oil yield, and then soaked in water.

REGIONS OF ORIGIN:
Brazil, Caribbean, Comoros Islands, India, Indonesia, Malaysia, Réunion, Sri Lanka.

CHARACTERISTICS:
Vetivert is a dark brown or amber viscous essential oil that easily drops from the bottle dropper.

FRAGRANCE DESCRIPTION:
Vetivert has deep, smoky, earthy top notes and sweet, musty, woody, potato undertones.

SAFE USAGE: Vetivert is a safe essential oil.

PLANT DESCRIPTION

Vetivert is a tall perennial grass.

BLENDING PROFILE

Vetivert blends well with sweet orange, mandarin, sweet marjoram, sandalwood, lemon, neroli, cardamom, rose, jasmine, lavender, ylang ylang, geranium, patchouli, and clary sage.

TRADITIONAL USES

In India, vetivert is grown to protect against soil erosion. In Ayurvedic medicine decoctions of vetivert are used to alleviate thirst, heatstroke, fever, and headaches. Vetivert is used to cool inflammatory disorders, and in the perfume industry.

THERAPEUTIC PROPERTIES

Antiseptic, antispasmodic, depurative, nervine, sedative, tonic, and vermifuge. *(See glossary on page 158.)*

Grounding and regenerating

Vetivert helps you find your tranquil center. Used in aftershave lotions and men's toiletries, vetivert is also recommended in baths, massage blends, and skin lotions. For women it can balance hormones during menopause. Overall, it is grounding, regenerating, and protecting.

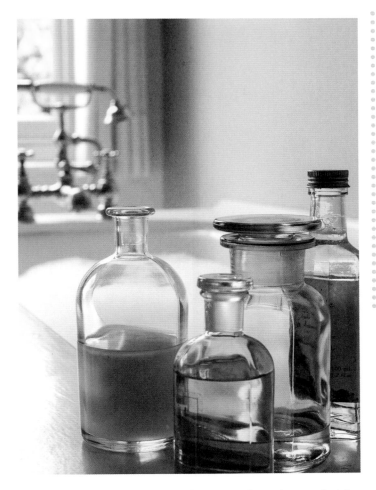

Vetivert is good in massage for muscular aches, arthritis, and rheumatism. It strengthens and tones tired, loose, and undernourished mature skin. Vetivert is an immuno stimulant, indicated when stress depletes the body's natural defenses.

Tones subtle energies

Psychologically, vetivert is valuable for nervous exhaustion, depression, anxiety, and insomnia. Calming, soothing, and restorative, vetivert tones subtle energies and balances the root chakra. It protects against over sensitivity, facilitating visionary insights, and wisdom.

Soothing bath soak

Whenever you feel exhausted, a bath with vetivert is deeply restorative. (Dispersant bath oil is a base oil that contains a dispersant, which allows the oils to mix into the water.)

You will need:

- tea-light candles
- 1 tsp dispersant bath oil
- 3 drops vetivert essential oil
- 1 drop lavender essential oil
- 2 drops neroli essential oil

1. Run a bath. Place tea-light candles nearby on a safe flat surface.

2. Light the candles, turn off electric light and, just before you get in, mix the oils and swish around in the water.

3. Climb in, lie back, and let go. Feel the tension and stress of the day slip away. As you enjoy the fragrance, notice each breath becoming longer and deeper as you relax, until you feel completely tranquil.

BENZOIN

Styrax benzoin

Botanical Family:
Styracaceae

Benzoin soothes, comforts, and elevates. It can also be used to drive away "evil spirits," or psychic exhaustion.

METHOD OF EXTRACTION:
Incisions into the bark produce resin "tears." The essential oil is steam distilled from these and then further dissolved in ethyl glycol.

REGIONS OF ORIGIN:
Cambodia, China, Indonesia, Laos, Malaysia, Sumatra, Thailand, Vietnam.

CHARACTERISTICS:
Benzoin is orange-brown, viscous, and sticky. Friar's balsam, a compound tincture of benzoin, is easier to use.

FRAGRANCE DESCRIPTION:
Benzoin has vanilla ice cream top notes and sweet molasses, balsamic undertones. Siam benzoin has a refined vanilla, chocolate note.

SAFE USAGE: Safe but can cause skin sensitization. Don't use in the bath; it leaves a yellow, sticky deposit.

PLANT DESCRIPTION

Benzoin is a tropical tree growing up to 65 feet high.

BLENDING PROFILE

Benzoin blends well with resin and spice oils, and also with rose, sandalwood, jasmine, cypress, juniper berry, lemon, and pine needles.

TRADITIONAL USES

Chinese herbalists used benzoin as a urinary tract antiseptic, a digestive aid, and for its heating and drying qualities. Burned as incense, benzoin is reputed to drive away evil spirits.

THERAPEUTIC PROPERTIES

Anti-inflammatory, antiseptic, astringent, carminative, deodorant, expectorant, sedative, and styptic. *(See glossary on page 158.)*

Valuable cold remedy

Benzoin's sweet fragrance comforts the sad, lonely, alienated, depressed, and bereaved. Benzoin and friar's balsam used in steam inhalations are valuable cold remedies, gentle enough for children. Benzoin treats asthma, bronchitis, and coughs. Overall, it is warming, soothing, and nurturing.

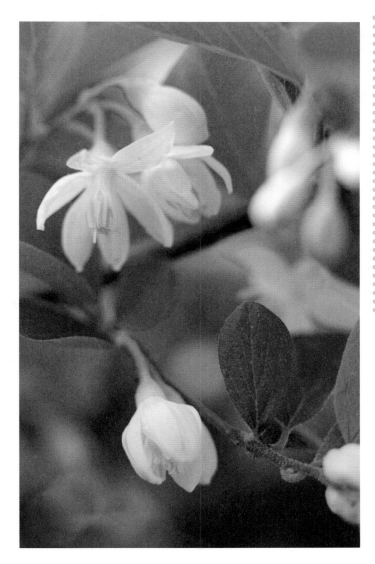

Hand cream

This hand cream is brilliant for cracked and chapped skin.

You will need:

- 1 x 2 fl oz (50 ml) dark glass jar
- 1½ oz (40 g) unfragranced base cream
- 2 tsp shea butter
- 1 tsp sweet almond oil
- 10 drops benzoin essential oil
- 5 drops myrrh essential oil

1. Spoon the cream into the jar.
2. Put the shea butter into a pyrex jug and stand in boiling water until melted.
3. Spoon the butter into the base cream and mix in quickly.
4. Stir in the sweet almond oil, benzoin, and myrrh until everything is well integrated.
5. Label the jar with ingredients, amounts used, and date.

Benzoin is useful in skincare, especially when skin is cut, chapped, cracked, or inflamed. It is good in massage blends for poor circulation and to relieve the pain of arthritis and rheumatism.

Chakra balancing
Psychologically, benzoin acts like a shield protecting you from the harshness of life. It helps balance heart and base chakras.

GLOSSARY

analgesic: relieves or diminishes pain

anaphrodisiac: relieves or diminishes sexual desire

anti-allergenic: relieves or reduces the symptoms of allergies

antibacterial/ antibiotic: prevents the growth of or destroys bacteria

anticatarrhal: relieves or reduces the production of mucus

anti convulsive: relieves or controls convulsions

antidepressant: uplifting and counteracting depression

anti-inflammatory: relieves or alleviates inflammation

antimicrobial: resists or destroys pathogens

antineuralgic: relieves or reduces nerve pain

antirheumatic: relieves or reduces the symptoms of rheumatism

antiseborrheic: helps control the products of sebum

antiseptic: destroys or controls pathogenic bacteria

antispasmodic: relieves spasms and cramps of smooth muscles

antisudorific: diminishes sweating

antitoxic: counteracts poisoning

antiviral: inhibits the growth of viruses

aphrodisiac: increases or stimulates sexual desire

astringent: contracts and tightens tissues

bactericidal/ bactericide: prevents the growth or destroys bacteria

balsamic: soothing and healing

carminative: settles the digestion, eases gripes and relieves flatulence

cephalic: stimulates and clears the mind

cholagogue: stimulates the flow of bile from the gall bladder into the intestines

cicatrizant: promotes healing by the formation of scar tissue

cytophylactic: stimulates the growth of healthy new skin cells

decongestant: relieves or reduces congestion, especially of mucus

demulcent: soothes, softens and alleviates irritation of the mucous membranes

deodorant: counteracts body odors

depurative: purifies and cleanses the blood

detoxifying: helps eliminate toxins from the body

digestive: aids the digestion of food

diuretic: increases the production and secretion of urine

emmenagogue: promotes and regulates menstruation

expectorant: helps expel mucus from the respiratory system

febrifuge: reduces fever

fungicidal/fungicide: resists or destroys fungal infections

galactagogue: increases the flow of breast milk

hemostatic: helps stop bleeding

hepatic: liver tonic, stimulates and aids liver function

hypertensor/ hypertensive: increases blood pressure

hypotensor/ hypotensive: reduces blood pressure

immunostimulant: stimulates the function of the immune system

insecticidal/ insecticide: destroys insects

laxative: aids bowel evacuation

nervine: nerve tonic, stimulates and strengthens the nervous system

rubefacient: warms the skin and increases blood flow

sedative: calms and reduces nervousness, distress and agitation

splenic: tonic of the spleen

stimulant: stimulates the physiological functions of the body

stomachic: tonic of the stomach and aids digestion

styptic: astringent, helps prevent external bleeding

tonic: invigorates and strengthens the body

uterine: tonic of the uterus

vasoconstrictor/ vasoconstrictive: constricts and contracts the capillary walls

vasodilator: causes dilation of the capillaries

vulnerary: promotes the healing of wounds, and prevents tissue degeneration

INDEX